Everything is in the process of being forgotten. But who we are—who we have been in mood, in personality, in character—persists much longer.

What gives her inner world cohesion is not thought but emotion.

Our relationship is changed now, but it is not yet ended. There is for us an opening, an opportunity that will be our last chance together.

I WANT TO REMEMBER

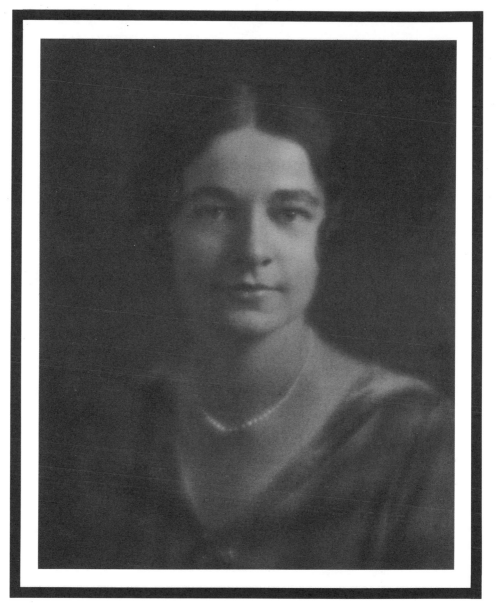

A SON'S REFLECTION ON HIS MOTHER'S
ALZHEIMER JOURNEY

•

DAVID DODSON GRAY

I WANT TO REMEMBER: *A Son's Reflection on His Mother's Alzheimer Journey.*

For information write to Roundtable Press, Four Linden Square, Wellesley, MA 02181.

Printed in the United States of America.

ISBN 0-934512-06-X

Library of Congress Catalog Card Number: 93-84913

Contents

Part 1.
Prelude

1.

Taking the Measure
of Alzheimer's Disease

It is nearly a year ago that my mother died. She lived with Alzheimer's disease for five years, and for her last two and a half years she was in a nursing home not far from where we live.

But what I have to tell is not mainly about the specifics of our experiencing together her Alzheimer's disease, for those details pertain only to her and to me. What I want instead to focus upon are elements which may be common to the experience of many of us who are one way or another involved with Alzheimer's disease.

"It's Not Over till It's Over"

One of the main things my mother and I learned from this experience is how meaningful it can be. A great many people throw up their hands and give up when someone becomes confused or forgetful and is diagnosed as "having Alzheimer's disease."

The problem with such a diagnosis is it sometimes becomes a terrible label, something that means there is no use trying any longer. That's simply not true, either for the patient or for their family.

Just because someone loses patience with themselves, they don't then have to lose hope and quit. And all too often people think because someone can't find the right word or can't always remember something they said (or that happened) five minutes ago, then that person isn't a real person any more.

That's simply not so.

Let me tell you a story which illustrates what I mean. Six or eight months before she died, my mother for weeks at a time wasn't able to say things that made any sense to me, so I took the initiative in more and more of our conversations. I had no idea whatsoever whether my mother was understanding what I was telling her, but I kept on talking to her as though she did. It was clear from her always alert eyes and her expression that she was enjoying my attention, whether she was really grasping my meaning or not.

There is for us an opening, an opportunity
that will be our last chance together.

By this time I was having to feed her, so much of my running commentary was about what she was eating, events in my day, the weather outside today, and the like. At various times I took to telling her what I hoped would be interesting highlights from the current news. The year was 1988 and an election year, and I told her, for example, that a black man named Jesse Jackson was running for president—and getting quite a few votes. To most of my capsule news summaries I got no response; she just kept on swallowing.

Then, after at least two weeks in which my mother had said nothing that I could understand in the least, one night I told her, "Mom, you may not know that there is a woman who is president in the Philippines. This weekend some of the military tried to force her out."

She continued taking my spoonfuls of food, chewing, swallowing. Another spoonful, chew, swallow. Suddenly and with crystal clarity she said to me in an almost whispery voice, "Did they get her?"

I was thrilled; I had gotten through to her—and she had been able to transmit back to me this message of reception, recognition, and response. And I reassured her, "Oh no, she is still president. The military tried, and failed."

My point in recounting this story is to make clear my mother's experience and my own that even after she seemed to have retreated very far within the isolation of Alzheimer's disease, she—the person who had been and still was my mother—was still present. She was not who she once had been, no—far from it. But there were these occasional moments when she could break through the constraints of the Alzheimer's and let me see her briefly again, her old fire now burning low but still going.

Life-Transformations

Experiences like this I found very meaningful, and I think my mother did too, for we both knew she was in big trouble. I am sure she had long since forgotten the Alzheimer's label and what it connoted. But she knew this was not the way her life was supposed to be.

What was happening to her (and to me through my involvement with her) was that my mother, like every Alzheimer's patient, was going through one of those few-in-a-lifetime life transformations that every few decades we all experience.

Everyone's first life-transformation is when we are born, separated from our mother's umbilical cord and uterus. In this and in each of the life transforming experiences that come later on, we find ourselves largely unprepared. We continue being who we were but we are being compelled to change rapidly. We have few or no experiences or resources to guide us. Those around us, if we are fortunate, are loving and caring and supportive. But we soon discover we are largely on our own, for they cannot do this living and coping for us.

Most of all in these times, each of us is on our own.

The greatest previous life transformation for many women is the experience of conception, pregnancy, child-birth and then mothering for the next 18 or 20 years. Nothing quite prepares a woman for this demanding and totally absorbing experience which demands more energy and endurance and sensitivity, and more intelligent problem-solving and accountability, than most mothers feel they are capable of. But, no matter, they are carried forward by the demands of this major life transformation and they must live ever afterwards with how well or how poorly they managed to do it. Their life is like a river filled with rapidly moving flood-waters carrying them along in its swift flow. The best they can do is learn to swim *with* rather than against the currents, trying to make the best of where they are carried by these life-forces of change.

Men, and women too, have an often similar life-transforming experience when they are let go from a job and don't find work for what seems like an eternity of looking, coping, learning, trying to adapt, always hoping to regain their financial stability, job satisfaction, and some sort of vocational stability. It is my impression that divorcing (or being divorced) also often has this same life-transforming character in which we seem to careen down a bumpy road moving swiftly, dangerously, out of control.

But in all of these experiences, as with Alzheimer's disease, our lives do not (at least yet) come to an end. The person we have been is uprooted, heavily stressed, fearful over losing so much control both of ourselves and of circumstances, and feeling not at our strongest or best. But we are still ourselves. Placid people are still placid, angry people are still angry, selfish people are still selfish, fearful people are still fearful. Personality or character persists amid life transformations and indeed shapes our response to such crises, affecting how other people respond to us and so affecting how things turn out. In my mother's all-Alzheimer unit of thirty-four patients in the nursing home, it was clear to me and also to the staff that Alzheimer's was much harder for some patients than for many others. It was no picnic for anyone, but some made it much harder by the way they were and how they approached life. "Mean people are still mean" was the way one very caring and perceptive staff member put it to me.

Assessing the "Pluses" That Go with Alzheimer's

I am fifty-nine now. My father died eighteen years ago of what today we would know as Alzheimer's disease. My mother had it. If there is any genetic link, I may well get it. Looking back (and looking ahead), what do I conclude?

In my years as an Episcopal minister I have been with a lot of people in their last years and months of life, and I really don't see that there is any easy way to die except suddenly—dropping in your tracks or in your sleep. Few of us are so fortunate.

As one older friend observed, "Growing old isn't for sissies." But that said, I really don't think Alzheimer's is so bad as it is cracked up to be. "How can I say that?" you ask. Two things come immediately to my mind.

The future for them was mercifully obscured along with the past.

My mother for many years had osteoporosis, the disease that results from calcium leaching out of the bones after menopause. The disks in her spine finally began to collapse and caused her intense shooting pain. This was about the time her Alzheimer's started to click in. As her Alzheimer symptoms increased in intensity, I noticed that my mother's spinal pain from her osteoporosis was overcome or removed. At least it wasn't an issue she ever again spoke about or seemed affected by. I noticed also among the fifty or sixty Alzheimer's patients I came to know over several years that I saw no hands swollen by arthritis or any indications of painful movements or joints.

So it seems to me that those with Alzheimer's are by and large spared a lot of the chronic physical pain that is the frequent accompaniment of old-age infirmity or cancer or dying. My observation is that nothing erodes well-being and morale so thoroughly as pain. Alzheimer's seems to represent a fork in the road of life for most and perhaps all. If you go with Alzheimer's, at least you are spared the mental and physical torment of many sorts of pain.

The other thing about Alzheimer's is that, along with all the confusion and disorientation, you seem to lose not only your sense of place on the spatial map but also your sense of place on the time-map of your own lifetime. Not only do you no longer know what town or city you are in but you have lost the imaginative capacity to imagine with anxiety and existential dread your own dying. My mother knew something was very wrong. She knew she really was not herself as she had for so long liked to be. But she was now incapable of experiencing the apprehensions of a cancer patient dreading a recurrence or, of a cancer patient later, simply wasting away and knowing the end is coming closer with each tick of some clock.

In common with cancer patients, my mother and her Alzheimer companions in the nursing home were also on a slippery slope from which there would finally be no escaping. But as they settled into their Alzheimer's disease, the future for them receded until they were living solely in the moment, the now. The future for them was mercifully obscured along with the past. Within the limits of their present moments of experience, my mother and her neighbors were able to enjoy not only the absence of chronic physical pain but also affectionate care, people who treated them with dignity and respect, and such pluses as music and color and good smells and little taste-treats. They formed friendships, enjoyed companionship, some women still flirted, men still took women for walks, women talked to women by the hour, and I gradually became aware that a gentle sensuality and eroticism still thrived. In short all of their lives continued as blurred but distinguishable continuations of who they had once been.

Alzheimer's Skills to Learn

The final thing I want to say is that I found there are definite skills we who are supportive caregivers or family can learn. When we cannot go on together as we have in the past, we who are not ill can learn new ways to continue many of the satisfactions of before. The Alzheimer's patient can't learn so readily as we can, so it is for us to do much of the adapting.

I am here to bear witness that there is more good living in the midst of Alzheimer's disease than doctors, or occasional visitors to patients, know how to see. There are many things about Alzheimer's patients that caring and sensitive staff can come to know as they live with them hour after hour. This is fortunate, both for patients and for their families. But as you will see in the following chapters, there are many other aspects to the inner life of Alzheimer's patients, recollections from all those now-gone good years we lived together. These bygone times the Alzheimer patient suddenly brings up like a relic from an archeological dig, and only family can know what to make of such clues from the past. Only family can imagine what these mean as we embark upon this journey together.

I am here to bear witness that
there is a lot more good living that goes on
in the midst of Alzheimer's disease
than doctors and occasional visitors
know how to see.

What we are going to discover here is as much about ourselves as it is about the one we love who has Alzheimer's disease. Our relationship with one another is changed now, but it is not yet ended. There is for us an opening, an opportunity that will be our last chance together. It can become a very meaningful new period in which we find new roles and finally come to terms with what our lives until now have meant.

So do not panic. Don't flee. This relationship is not over yet. This will not be easy but it need not be the worst thing that ever happened to you. In considerable measure it is up to you, as the healthy one here, to define what you will bring to this situation. You will set the limits to what you and the Alzheimer patient can get out of this period in both your lives.

Finally, all this will not go on forever. It will end in probably a thousand or two thousand days. So take these days one at a time. You can do it. Give a little to these days and you can get a lot. Try it. See.

2.

The Roaring in My Ears

I was sitting with my mother while she ate her supper. True to form, she had started with the cookies. She broke one and shared it with me. "Boys always like cookies," she observed, although anyone my age can scarcely remember what it was like to be a boy. But I guess that to mothers their sons always remind them of the boys we once were. At least it was so this night.

We were talking lightly back and forth about our respective days, my mother interspersing her comments with garble-garble now and then. But this was one of her more lucid times, or so I thought until she picked up her fork and dipped it into her milk glass like a soup spoon. She then brought it carefully to her mouth and was a little surprised it was empty.

Her world these days seems to me like that, so filled with such surprises. Things she would anticipate working out one way actually turn out some other way. She tries to say one thing and something else comes out, a garble. Or she gets half-way into a thought and suddenly has lost her way. I have done that too. I call it "losing my train of thought." But her experiences are more frequent and more ultimate because much of the time what she starts out toward suddenly evaporates, is gone.

There was a period when this forgetting in mid-thought bothered her and she was frustrated by it. Then later she was simply embarrassed by it if others than immediate family were there. But now she simply rides her underlying streams of emotions as though she were the empress being given a personal tour on her own inflated raft through white-water rapids, down the Colorado River and the Grand Canyon.

On and on it goes, day after day, and she seems to have found some happy elixir of age which lets her feel that the waters right around her are somehow calmed, for as far as I can see the waters splash and churn and rage in an excitement approaching terror. All I can think of is my own adolescent experiences riding the roller coaster at Canobie Lake, New Hampshire. But she is as nice and as gracious about it as if she were serving you tea and her own warm apple pie on a tablecloth at her mother's kitchen table. I wonder if I will have those sorts of emotional resources when the waters rage about me, if I get to her years.

I wonder what our generation is going to do
when finally it's our turn to be
where they are now.

I was talking on the phone the other day with a colleague, a woman who went to my wife's college and who first raised a family before becoming now a minister in a nearby town. Her father has Alzheimer's too. Her mother is caring for her father, and she is keeping an eye on them both. "And the money goes out in big chunks day after day," she observed.

"I wonder what our generation is going to do when finally it's our turn to be where they are now," I mused. It's a thought I find more and more on the minds of our fifties age-group.

For the past several years my wife and I have been receiving from our alma maters, Smith College and Yale, glossy four-color mailing pieces that advertise tours for alums to exotic and remote places. We have realized that some of our number now have both the time and the means to go for three weeks to China or for two and a half weeks on a square rigger on the Caspian Sea (or something equally exotic.)

While we were all raising our children, almost everyone we know did not have very much money for extras. What we are realizing now is that some of us did not have much money then because we were in occupations called "human services" but which back then were simply teaching and the ministry and all the other Good Samaritan callings that every society needs. Such occupations are big on psychic satisfactions, and yield extremely modest incomes. We always told ourselves we weren't doing it for the money.

We are realizing finally that some among us did not have very much money for extras back then because each pay period they were making more and socking a lot of it away in anticipation of the proverbial rainy days. Those rainy days are finally coming. Like us they see them coming too. And they are getting in their trips and other extravagances while the getting is good. I think we would too, if we could.

My colleague is very honest: "Sometimes Jack and I wonder what we would do if either of us lost our jobs. We'd be out on the street in about three months." Those same thoughts have crossed our minds too. I'm sure they have crossed the minds of a lot of people in our society, not just today but in many generations past. But in our time we have the potential, the capacity (with luck) to live so long. We would not at all change the lives we have lived and the work we have done. We know society needs this sort of work. But it is just that it won't pay for it very well. Being old can be very expensive. My mother doesn't worry about that any more; I do, for her and for us.

So even before we feel the spray of the rapids in our own faces, we can hear the roar in our ears of those waves, those rapids ahead. Someday we will be trying to eat milk with a fork and not worrying. Well, all I can do today is be a companion to my mother, share her cookies with her and be her boy. That too is something society needs of us all, and we owe to one another. But somehow it got left out of the cash-and-income economy.

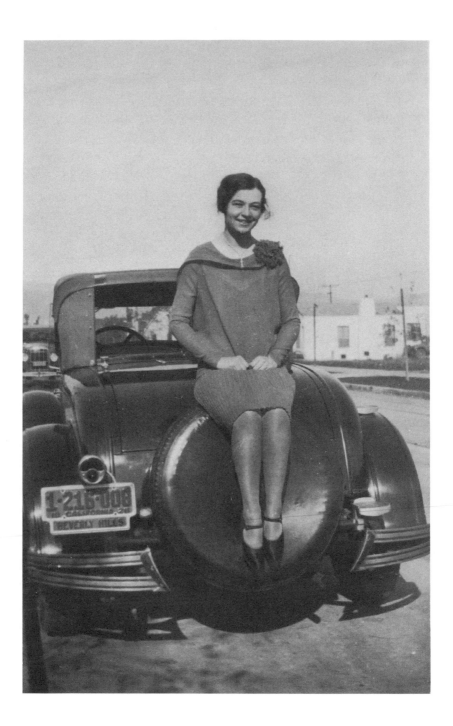

Part 2.
The Long March

Opposite page: The Roadster, 1928, Beverly Hills.

3.

Early Winter's Dusk

The Cold Chill

The sun is setting as I walk in the winter's cold the half-mile from our house to the nursing home. It is a walk of memories and of chilled testing, for the way to visiting my mother is across the open playing fields of the Junior High and, as the sun slowly settles behind the bare tree limbs, any warmth that there was in the winter's day is quickly gone and the wind sweeps strongly as though straight out of Ontario and Hudson Bay's deepest winter-cold.

Each day I set out, bundled against outer cold and ready to enjoy the invigorating briskness of this winter's walk and the warm haven at the end of it. Some nights I could walk further and the end comes quickly, while other nights the wind is so fierce and penetrating I can scarcely wait to get inside again. The nursing home is always warm, overly warm, and I look forward to that welcoming contrast and to a few more last hours with my mother. These times have been precious for some months and we both have known it.

"There you are," she greets me, "how've you been?" "Fine," I tell her, taking her hand. "Your hand's cold," she tells me. "It's cold outside," I say, "but I'll warm up in a minute—How's your day gone?"

"I didn't catch that," I say. "Say it again."

"Oh," I say, "that's interesting. Did you like that?" I am responding to the inflection of her voice because the syllables are garbled with sometimes a word or a string of words I can use as signposts. But the territory is like an unfamiliar city at night when the streets look all alike, strange, and there are too few street signs and directions.

I catch the name of neighbors across the street ten and twenty-five years ago. "Oh, you've been thinking of the Wises today; I haven't thought of them in years." More garble. "They were good neighbors, weren't they." Garble, a few more words, more garble. "He's gone now, isn't he, and I suppose she is too." Garble.

I am responding to the inflection of her voice because the syllables are garbled with sometimes a word or a string of words I can use as signposts. But the territory is like an unfamiliar city at night when the streets look all alike, strange, and there are too few street signs and directions.

That reminds me of Pop Kriegal. "I haven't thought of him in years either," I say. "What was his daughter's name?" My mother tells me and I recognize she's right—and I quickly forget because Pop Kriegal's daughter's name is no longer important to me. "That was a good neighborhood for you and Dad, wasn't it," I say.

By now Mom has warmed my hand in her own, her eyes are bright with relatedness and interest and involvement in our conversation and our time together. It is another precious moment for us both, her son is here with her and I am able to be with my mother again. I know such times are slipping from us in the same way the last grains of sand slip through the neck of an hourglass. This life's clock is getting close to its midnight, some bell will soon chime and it will be tolling not for me but for my mother. And then, like the fairy-tale account of Cinderella's coach at the grand ball, suddenly this life will turn from being a crystal coach bearing this princess and suddenly become a pumpkin, broken, shattered, only a remnant of its former glory. My mother's hand is still warm in mine and now my hand is warming her's.

Remembered Warmth

"Your hand is cold, are you warm enough?" I ask. "Oh, yes, thank-you. How was your day?" she asks. She is good at these routine pleasantries. She has always known how to be interested and draw us out, for she really was interested in how her children and grandchildren were doing, what they were up to, what interesting tidbits about them we could bring. I start to tell her about our day, the mail, the book orders, the phone calls, the plans for our next speaking trip. We'll be going to Seattle and then we are thinking of a quick side trip to the new Expo in Vancouver. I re-live with her some of our previous trips, and colleagues at the University of British Columbia whom she has never met but whose existence has always vaguely interested her, reassuring her (as it does me) that what we do is of some worth, some significance and social contribution. "Then," I continue, "we may be able to come home by way of San Diego and see our daughter. Yes, Lisa is in Southern California now, at about the same age you were when your parents lived in Beverly Hills."

There are some moments of lucid recall about those years when she was twenty-four and soon to be married to my father. She and her sister and a friend spent part of a winter in California in 1928. Her father got them a roadster, my mother danced the Charleston, and it was all very gay and young and fun. "Isn't it amazing to think that Lisa is now that age and there with her young man just as you were?" We bask in that retrospective moment and we both enjoy the implied accomplishment of being old enough to have your grandchildren recapitulate some aspects of your own life in a same but very different world. My mother smiles a wise and deeply satisfied smile, "And what about you?" she asks.

In the background of our conversation I am aware of another patient, not my mother's eighty-two but closer to my own age, fifty-five or sixty. She is reaching over, she is taking the emptied can which had contained my mother's favorite supper for many years, a can of Ensure nutritional supplement. Louise is emptying it into her own glass; there is only a trickle. My mother and I talk on, and a few minutes later Louise, having forgotten the previous moment but still apparently thirsty, reaches over again and tries once more to find something in the still empty can. A few minutes later the efforts are repeated again. The phonograph needle is stuck and repeats itself; the groove of memory is worn out except for the present moment. Alzheimer's steals not only the future, it steals the past. My mother and I continue to bask in the emotional warmth of the moment. The fire in our relationship is dimming but we huddle close. We are together and we treasure it, both of us knowing there is not a lot more.

The phonograph needle is stuck and repeats itself;
the groove of memory is worn out
except for the present moment.

I am outside again, and the long dusk of early winter has finally gone into night. The wind is at my back going home and I am melancholy. There is a sadness in this time of winter's dusk when all the trees, stripped bare, are outlined against the sky, lit from behind by light from a sun which has already slipped beyond the seen horizon. But now the dusk is gone and the chill of night is settling in, and that is worse. The light is gone and my feet crunch dry and cold upon the frozen grass. Moved by the wind at my back I am quickly at my door and I suddenly re-enter the familiar world of another generation, my own. I am again inside where it is warm, there is dinner to help prepare, and I call to my Liz, "I'm home, what can I do?"

We move together in a familiar pattern in our kitchen as I tell her of the cold and of the warmth and of my mother's bright intensity, the pleasure in her eyes and the glint of her emotion as we talked of old neighbors and of grandchildren. I knew that tomorrow for Mom would be another blank slate upon which she would try to write, and I would hold her warm hand once or twice or a few times more. But the bright sun's warmth was gone from our days and its light was slipping beyond our horizon. This winter dusk is long and cold and precious still.

4.

Ghosts

I Live among Ghosts

Those I see nearly every day who have Alzheimer's disease are ghosts, for today they are mere apparitions of who they once were. My mother is a ghost.

One of the most prominent features of Alzheimer's disease is the steady loss of memory. You forget names. You can't find the word you want. But then it gets worse and goes beyond this familiar and everyday experience we all have known. You lose your way in familiar places. You lose track of time—the time of day, the season, the year, how old you are, and so on. My mother is seventy-nine if you ask her, though chronologically she is nearly eighty-three. She even forgets now that she forgets. That is how it is with Alzheimer's disease.

Diamonds in This Quicksand

Forgetting that she forgets turns out to be a blessing as well as being a source of confusion. "Why didn't someone tell me that?" she has asked me upon occasion. "We did tell you," I respond, "but a part of your illness is that you forget." "Oh yes," she'll muse, for she has even forgotten that she has this dread affliction. I am glad she can forget she has Alzheimer's disease and that she doesn't have to hold that worry up to herself continually as if it were a mirror in which she was always seeing herself.

My own experience with my mother and her companions in this special-care unit for Alzheimer's patients is that there are amazing blessings for them even amid their great adversities. For example, what they are losing is their memories, their memories of how to tie their shoes, how to dress themselves, and they forget sooner or later how to hold their urine, how to feed themselves, even how to walk and their own names. Everything, it seems, is in the process of being forgotten.

But who they are—who they have been in mood, in personality, in character—persists much longer. How long, I haven't the experience yet to say. But it is longer, considerably longer.

I am glad she can forget she has
Alzheimer's disease and that she doesn't have to
hold that worry up to herself continually
as if it were a mirror
in which she was always seeing herself.

What this means for my mother and her companions is that relationships among them do develop, albeit without our usual capacities for conversation. At first I did not understand that this was happening. It seemed to me, back then, that they were simply talking past one another and were completely unmindful that what they had just said was in no way a reply.

But I have come to see that, far from being unmindful of what is going on around them, my mother and many of her companions seem hyperalert. You and I have learned to tune out what we regard as background noises and background conversations. What we are attending to is for us "foreground," and everything else is "background." The background is what needn't concern us. But my mother now hears all of that and seems intent upon responding to whatever she can understand. It doesn't matter to her any longer that the conversation is outside in the hall. Or is taking place across the common room (where she and her neighbors in the unit spend most of their time). Or is taking place at the nursing station not far from her room. It is all "foreground" for her.

My mother and I can be talking in her room in that hour late in the afternoon which is after her supper but before mine. It is a time when there is considerable coming and going outside but near her room. She and I will have something going between us, with each of us enjoying responding to the other. And then suddenly she is talking, responding to something from another world, the world outside her room. "Come in," she may call out. Or "I don't know, but maybe." She feels responsible and responds to it all.

You and I have learned to tune out
what we regard as background noises
and background conversations. . . .
It is all "foreground" for her.

Like Ladies of the Club

So when my mother and her companions sit at a mealtime around a circular table for four, there is not what you and I think of as conversation. It seemed to me like crazy-talk at first, a garble of words and syllables that seems most of the time to be sheer nonsense. But as I participate in it more regularly, I realize that their time together has much in common with women's talk over a bridge game or at a church gathering where women are sewing and talking. They are passing the time together, being nice to each other (usually) but with no heavy conversation. It is what we used to call "chatting."

Last evening is an example. My mother was finishing her supper and I was sitting with her when a woman whose name I haven't mastered yet wheeled up in her wheelchair. I have spoken to this woman many times as she was laboriously exercising by wheeling her chair back and forth from nowhere to nowhere. She clearly has a heavy mood and has had what I take to be a difficult life. But last night she wheeled up to us and clearly wanted to join in the pleasantries of our conversation.

My mother reached out to touch the woman's knee and garbled to her some syllables and words I could not make out. But the woman responded immediately, saying—"I'm going home soon, are you going home? My mother's there and my sister."

My reaction was amazement at how ungarbled her words and sentences were, for my mother's talk was much more disintegrated. But my mother returned this opening gambit and replied, "Your sister—."

"Yes, my sister. You know her—Mrs. Gordon."

Somewhere out of the sunny recesses of my mother's disposition she supplied a single word—"Beautiful." Her companion immediately picked up on that and was agreeing, "Yes, my sister is really beautiful." Any sisterly rivalries about beauty seemed long gone; I am sure her mother is long gone too. She was disoriented about where she was and when in her life she was, but in many other respects she could function quite well. My mother was much more absent and less herself.

The conversation went on, my mother now and again providing a word or phrase that was vaguely appropriate as a response. Her companion was able to provide the substance and much of the flow and progression of the conversation she clearly wanted to have.

"Who's your doctor?" she asked. I was sure this was her form of padding the conversation with stuff she felt comfortable with. But it was clearly asking more of my mother than my mother could provide. She reached for a last sip of her milk, sipped it, and then began rearranging the plates and cutlery on her tray.

I have seen many conversations like this. And not all of them in nursing homes, mind you. But those of us who are not patients seem more attuned to these lapses of continuity when we are among relatives and colleagues with Alzheimer's disease. Somehow we see these ghostlike traits more clearly there.

Alzheimer's disease produces
effects that are like a
jostled phonograph needle which "skips" or
"skids" into some other moment or place.

But all of us have times when we are not completely present to each other, times when we are groping for some strategy to ease our way (or another's way) through a momentary anxiety. And it is then that we "skid" a little, just the way a phonograph needle does when inadvertently we jostle the turntable. The needle skips to another groove and, if we are listening, we know we missed something in the continuity of the music, a few measures, a few notes, a few phrases. Alzheimer's disease produces effects like that jostled phonograph needle which skips or "skids" into some other moment or place.

"Can't You See I'm Busy?"

There is frequently occasion for humor in all this. I am not clear whether those with Alzheimer's are aware of it or not. I can't recall any of them laughing at some of the things their condition brings to pass.

I recall one particular evening in the common room. My mother and most of her neighbors were still sitting around the dinner tables in their chairs or wheelchairs. A few were sitting on the sofa by the piano, a few more in the tall-backed armchairs around the perimeter of the room. At this hour the radio or phonograph is usually on, or the television with the evening news.

The "walkers" were up and walking, as they often are. The four or so walkers amaze me. They spend all their free time exercising by walking. They act like they were former postal workers. One of the nursing supervisors told me they once put a pedometer on Sophie's ankle to measure how far she walked. They were amazed to find she had walked 17.2 miles in one day. So the walkers like Sophie and Adele and Bill really do walk, even amid the confines of this special care unit and the adjacent unit through the fire doors, where there is a more general population of older people who are now completely confined to their beds.

So the walkers move up and down these hallways, through the fire doors (if they can still manage that), walking, walking. On most evenings Sophie and Adele are among the walkers, and like schoolgirls they often walk hand in hand. But this particular night something was amiss between them.

I had been there but a short time so I hadn't seen the genesis of it. All I knew was that suddenly Adele was telling off her friend in a loud voice and wanting to separate their schoolgirl handclasp which Sophie wanted to maintain.

Adele now had her hand free. And suddenly in this place of infinite leisure I heard coming out of the mouth of this older woman the words of an exasperated schoolgirl: "Leave me alone, can't you see I'm *busy?*" And with that she turned on her heel (as rapidly as she could manage at her age) and walked off alone.

The whole exchange took place in a momentary lull after supper as they were standing by the doorway of the common room. Some of the others looked up, some did not. But quickly the sounds of voices and music and evening TV programming again dominated the room. Sophie then walked off by herself.

A little later as I was leaving, I saw them walking together, again hand in hand. The thought occurred to me that one of the blessings of Alzheimer's was that their earlier exchange had simply been forgotten. Or had they simply patched things up, as schoolgirls do?

In any event the soft pulse of life in the special care unit throbbed ever on.

"Anyone Here from CONOCO–DuPont?"

Another of my favorite ghosts is Ed Fitzgerald. Ed is a former New York banker. He has the carriage still of the important person he has recently been. He is tall, distinguished looking, with lovely flowing hair that is now completely white. Apart from his memory problems he looks much the same as many of his age-cohort who still are working out of the executive suites in the major banks of the City's financial district.

It is clear to me that Ed loved his work and misses it still. Part of this is that he is one of only five or six males in a unit with a capacity of thirty-four beds. He is surrounded by women. Ed is not an ardent walker but after dinner he quite frequently strolls about in the common room, asking aloud (half to himself, half to anyone who will listen), "Anyone here from Commercial Credit?" and then a few moments later or a few minutes later he will ask again, "Anyone from CONOCO–DuPont?"

> Much that Ed has found very dear is still the present content of his consciousness and concerns. "Who you have been is still who you are." But his capacity to remember it all is deteriorating faster for Ed than it is for the rest of us.

It is clear to me that like everyone else in the Alzheimer's unit, Ed brought with him his own mental world of experiences. It is increasingly garbled now but it is still the world he would like to talk and think about, the world of business and corporate finance that for so long focused his interest and fascination.

I was sitting with my mother last night and talking with her, when Ed shuffled over and sat down next to Sophie. She was resting for a moment before walking some more. She said something (I forget what). Ed's response was very much in character and also a complete non sequitur: "I'll tell you about CONOCO–DuPont."

Like many others here, Ed's Alzheimer's disease is causing him to be losing a lot of memories in a steadily progressing process. But over the four months I've known Ed as a neighbor of my mother, I have seen that there is also much which is not lost, at least not lost yet. Much that Ed has found very dear is still the present content of his consciousness and concerns. "Who you have been is still who you are." But his capacity to remember it all is deteriorating faster for Ed than it is for the rest of us. He is simply becoming a ghost faster than we are.

Ghosting

I find I am enjoying these times with my mother. She isn't the same person I knew a year, or five years, ago. But she wasn't then the person I had known as my mother when I was a young adult or when I was a child of school-age. She has changed with the years and so have I.

But I find her pleasure in my visits is consistent over the years. She is still interested in hearing about my day and whatever gossip I may have to bring about more distant members of the family. I must be honest and tell you that I do not know what she makes of much of what I tell her. But then I am sure I *never* knew all of her reactions. What has changed is her capacity to maintain, as fully as she used to, her part of the fabric of our back-and-forth relationship. More of that now falls to me.

I find that in order to enjoy her company (and to enjoy her pleasure in my company), more and more of the initiative and creativity has to be coming from my side of the relationship. It is a process we have seen with our own children when they were very small. And I know my mother went through it with me.

Every parent who does parenting as a mother-in-residence does, has done a lot of this "pumping up" of a relationship. We do it when the other one is too small and young (or in my mother's case, too old and mentally frail) to make it a symmetrical relationship among equals.

I find that in order to enjoy her company
(and to enjoy her pleasure in my company),
more and more of the initiative and creativity has to
be coming from my side of the relationship.

Parents do this when they talk to and take an interest in a very young child who cannot talk back. Later we do it when we spend time visiting parks and zoos with our children rather than dragging them, bored stiff and whining, through museums or cathedrals (or what-have-you) that would really interest us. Instead we select contexts for all of us to share together, contexts that will be safe and satisfying for everyone.

The difference is that with my mother I am aware the shoe is now, so to speak, on the other foot. I am the one who is moving life and our relationship along, just as when I was a child she did this for me. More than that, I realize she has done it in varying degrees and distances throughout our lives together—my entire lifetime.

So now the immediacy of her life and friendship and presence literally fades day after day from us both, and I name what we are doing together "ghosting." It is what we do with the people we care about and who have cared and nurtured us, as they fade from this mortal scene. We have a little time left, and ghosting is an extended form of reaching after their departing apparition as it slips from us. When death comes among us abruptly and one of us departs suddenly from good health, those who remain alive do this reaching, reaching, reaching after the other during the months that follow, as our memories gradually heal. As with a physical amputation, we are missing what is now lost.

But for those of us whose close relatives have Alzheimer's disease, we do our reaching while they are physically still among us. Their ghosts are here for a while and, with some effort, we can enjoy them still. They will be gone soon enough, but we can be saying our good-byes now. We have the unusual task (and privilege) of doing our ghosting among the living who—more obviously than the rest of us—we can see are on their way to being dead.

5.

Listening to Garble

Slipping

My brother was with me for this visit to my mother. I come nearly every day but his being here was special. He lives a thousand miles away and it has been a year—no, more like a year and a half—since he and our mother have seen one another.

For a time they were able to talk on the phone. But gradually that became less and less satisfying for both of them. More and more Mom was reaching for words and could not find them. She could listen but she could not react as she once had. There was less and less initiative she could take in the conversation. She loved hearing from him as she did from everyone.

But I became aware that she knew what was happening to their phone conversations and she was embarrassed by it. We were both on the line talking long-distance with her sister. They had not talked to one another in some time and I was prepared (as I am sure Aunt Mil was) to settle in for a prolonged chat. Suddenly my mother was saying, "Well, it's so nice to have talked to you." I realized she was trying to close off the conversation. Why?—I thought; she is feeling inadequate, can't remember, some words are escaping her, and she would rather not talk and would flee the contact rather than feel the anxiousness about how she is doing talking to her sister.

That time I computed all this quickly enough and, a rare thing for me, I overrode her will and said something she could respond to easily. She recovered and we all three could go on and have more contact, more conversation. But it was her last talk with her sister. A year earlier Mil and her husband had visited Mom at home for half an hour when they were in town for the graduation of their grandson from college. But we all knew Mom was "slipping," as that generation puts it. My brother's visit reimpressed that upon us both.

It is like the old radio transmissions when the
signal is weak or unclear
or filled with extraneous static—"garble."

"How's Your Day Been?"

Because I was seeing Mom so much, I was still a very familiar and welcome figure in her life. I appear regularly, I pull a chair over close by her, take her hand, and then I ask her, "How's your day been?" But I know much of what I will hear from her now is garble. It is like the old radio transmissions when the signal is weak or unclear or filled with extraneous static—"garble."

Then, as now, I knew I would have to listen intently to the flow amid the garble. A few words and sentence fragments come clear, or seem to. Sometimes a possible context seems to appear, giving me some possible clue to what remote part of her past or present she is now hooked into and ruminating about. Sometimes it is only the inflection in her voice at the end of a garbled sequence that gives me a clue that this is a question.

I respond to inflections suggesting a question the best I can. I have learned not to ask her to repeat something again; that is now long since impossible. But I can always move with the flow, helping her unfold even the confusion she is experiencing, hoping that again as has happened in the past, I will be able to clamber for a few moments with her onto the "raft" of the present moment as it moves swiftly in the rapidly moving stream of consciousness which is her inner world.

Sometimes there is a name, a word, something that locates us. Once it was just the name of "Mr. Scott," a next-door neighbor of long ago. A query and that cue enabled me to launch into a sympathetic reminiscence about what good neighbors the Scotts had been. "He must be gone now," I mused. "Yes, he's gone," she said completely clearly; this was a topic that brought lucid responses, which I took to mean that it was a topic close to her now. That made sense to me, emotional sense; I knew I'd be having thoughts and feelings about that in a situation like hers.

"George Baxter must be gone as well," I went on, "he was nearly Karl's age, ninety-two, when we last knew him." George Baxter had lived nearby and been cared for lovingly by a considerably younger wife.

"Karl's gone," my mother replied; Karl was her beloved older cousin and she came to help care for him after both their spouses died and Karl needed her. She had lived with Karl for a decade. But now at ninety-two himself, Karl was going strong compared with Mom.

"No," I said, "Karl's not gone. He just can't come see you in the nursing home because of his back problems; he can't drive that far in the car. He loves you very much, though, even if he can't come and see you."

"Oh," said Mom pensively. It was clear she had been thinking about Karl, thinking he too was "gone." Clearly that was a worry of hers and she had been grieving him. She was relieved even by the idea of his still being a part of this life despite the fact she was not going to see him.

I moved with the flow: "He would come to see you if he possibly could," I said. I tried to go further. "So many people have gone that it is hard to remember who has not," I said. "Yes" she said. "But you forget that you forget things, and that makes it harder." "Yes,"

Mom said. "It's hard not to worry about that," I said. "Yes," she said and squeezed my hand.

I forget what else we went on to talk about that night, but such moments of communication and recognition are precious. Like having tired feet gently rubbed, it doesn't change the situation but you do feel better for experiencing it. And I feel better for having been able to reach through the garble and get to my mother in the midst of her confused flow of thought-fragments and concerns.

The Excitement of a Visit from a Familiar Stranger

My brother's coming excited our mother a great deal. I had been making a point to tell her anew of his coming for each of the four days before. Each time was a new beginning with no sense from her of remembering she had ever heard that idea before. But when he and I came into her room, she knew this was special.

It has become clear to me that when she is feeling at ease and not anxious about a visitor making an adverse judgment about her or her condition, she has a lot on her mind she wants to share, to express.

It was not clear to my brother (or to me) whether she recognized him or ever became clear who he was. In our conversations about Rick coming she had shifted quickly to talking about "Mother," which in retrospect I realized sounded a lot like "brother." When he was there in her room, she held his hand warmly, her eyes twinkled as he kissed her and I pulled up the chair for him to sit close by her. I had greeted her saying, "I have Rick with me today, my brother," but soon she was talking about "Bill," whose only association for all of us is with our cousin, Mil's son, who lives (and has lived for twenty years) in Los Angeles.

Because she was excited, I thought, the garble has gotten heavier. This is confusing to our mother and, I thought, it is confusing to us. It must have been very confusing to my brother. Why, I wondered, is there all this about a "Bill"?

Suddenly, it fit. "You saw Bill when Aunt Mil was here in June for young Billy's graduation." Yes, that was it. They too had come from a long distance; the association made sense. My mother was too excited and disjointed either to confirm or deny it. Sometimes garble is like that; you think you may discern a meaning in it, you act on it, but you have to go on without confirmation from "the other side."

What gives her inner world cohesion is emotion. Garble is about emotion.

I was aware my brother, less familiar with our mother in this condition, was working to make sense of her garble but was finding it difficult. Not surprising, for this was to him a foreign language and new to him. I suggested to Mom that we were going to leave now, but we would both be coming back to see her again after her supper and before she went to bed. "You're coming back," she said. "Yes," we said. We kissed her, she kissed back, and we left.

Like Looking at Oneself in a Broken Mirror

Going down the stairs and then outside in the car we talked about Mom and about garble. "You hear things in all that which I don't," he said. "I just try to move with her emotional flow," I said. "I often can't understand the particulars. What I've called garble actually is a flow of words, of syllables, of phrases. It's like a computer which is dumping onto its printer a strange array of letters and numbers from somewhere. It is a configuration I don't know how to read, a garble."

"But," I told him, "I listen to the emotions." Some days recently she has been quite mellow, and I come in, pull up the chair, take her hand, and she is off and running. Those days she is the tour guide and I am the passive one. Those days I enjoy the ride, simply saying the appropriate things even when I don't quite understand.

Mom will go on, I notice, and interject what for her are certain stock phrases, her disclaimers of complete knowledge. She will garble something, and then say: "I think that's so, but maybe not." Or she will say something, and then ask me, "Isn't that so, or isn't it?—I don't know." There is endless variation on these themes, for it has become clear to me that when she is feeling at ease and unanxious about a visitor making an adverse judgment about her or her condition, she has a lot on her mind she wants to share, to express.

Like all of us, I think, she is seeking confirmation for her perceptions of reality. It must feel perhaps like looking in a broken mirror, all fragments and not any longer an integrated whole. Emotions matter now more than words and abstractions, and I have noticed she is drawn to them. On weekends the activities day of the unit is foreshortened and she watches television, especially sports. The emotional hype of a football announcer really draws her, the boxing announcer, the call of a horse race. Golf, bowling, the quieter-paced events, might as well not be happening. What gives her inner world cohesion is emotion. Garble is about emotion.

Sometimes the garble makes no sense (to me) but I sense in it the emotion of a question. "I really don't know about that," I say, making a more profoundly truthful statement than my mother realizes, "maybe so." Other times I'll say, "Could be, but I wouldn't know." I realize, midthought, that I am playing the garble back to her, reflecting my own indeterminacy in response to hers. "Say some more," I say, "I'd like to know more about it." Garble, garble. "Is that so!"—I comment, "of course." I realize that, like my mother earlier, I have learned to hide my lack of comprehension behind such stock words. But such words do help, they allow us to get on from moment to moment.

Getting beyond Our Longing for Clarity

One thing that bothers my brother, I realize, is that Mom's garble has alerted in him a response to confusions of reality which is widely held, namely, the need to understand *more* precisely rather than less. But amid all this garble from Alzheimer's disease, it is simply futile to try to get greater clarity about any one thing. It is like trying to bottle wind; there is no way you can do it.

One thing that bothers my brother, I realize, is that Mom's garble has alerted in him a response to confusions of reality which is widely held, namely, the need to understand *more* precisely rather than less.

I have concluded that trying to "see" amid garble is like one's trying to see at night. Have you ever noticed that at night you cannot see more clearly by simply trying to look more closely in our usual daytime ways? Instead we see best in the dark with the parts of our eyes that we cannot focus, the parts that pick up the wider picture. Listening to garble is like that kind of night vision. We often can see context even when we cannot see particulars. We might like details brought into greater clarity of expression and focus, but frequently the Alzheimer's patient cannot accommodate us.

My brother and I came back just before my mother would be getting ready for bed. It was clear she knew she had seen us earlier, that we had gone and now we had come back. We saw her for another fifteen minutes. This time she was much less excited, my brother was a much more familiar sight, and her garble was less.

I still did much of the talking. He held her hand and she his, and they looked a lot at each other as she talked. I think we all knew this was a very special time together, perhaps a last time. We did not have any "moment of silence," in memory of all the times we had ever had that were now past. My mother could no longer think thoughts like that. But my brother and I could, and for us that memory and emotion was so palpable it *was* the reality of that moment—for my brother and myself, if not for our mother.

We realized this separation now taking place, this slipping away. It was not clear then (or now) who was slipping away from whom. But the mother of our childhood was clearly long gone, or we were long gone from her. We gathered now in honor of the boys we had once been, the mother she once was, and in honor of the ties alive in us still between that long ago and who we all were now. We kissed again and left. She went to bed, we to dinner.

It was almost over. Except the garble. And the final curtain which had not yet fallen between us. It would soon go down. I would be back tomorrow and tomorrow and tomorrow. I felt not only like a son but like the man at the stage door waiting with flowers in his hand. The great star had already left the stage, and soon she would be leaving her dressing room. Forever.

6.

The Fragrance

"You Don't Need Birthdays Any More?"

My mother's eighty-second birthday was approaching. I had already bought for her a lovely floral card, but at this point in her life she is a difficult person to buy a present for.

Each day's visit with her heightens my awareness of how simpler her needs are. What she needs and delights in now are companionship, love, physical care and comfort. Perhaps, I muse, these and the card are enough.

Then a small package arrived, a gift from her younger sister Mil. I held the package for several days before bringing it to my mother. My thought is that I will spread out the celebration of Mom's birthday to allow her several days to savor it, and also to allow time for its happening to sink in. Earlier that week I mentioned to her several times that her birthday was coming soon. But I got no sign from her that she realized this or even that we had talked of it before.

"You don't need birthdays any more?" I asked her. She smiled.

Six months earlier when she had been entering the nursing home my mother responded to the social worker's question by saying she was seventy-nine. My sense at the time was that this must have been how old Mom was the last time her age made an impression on her. She made the same response about her age several other times too.

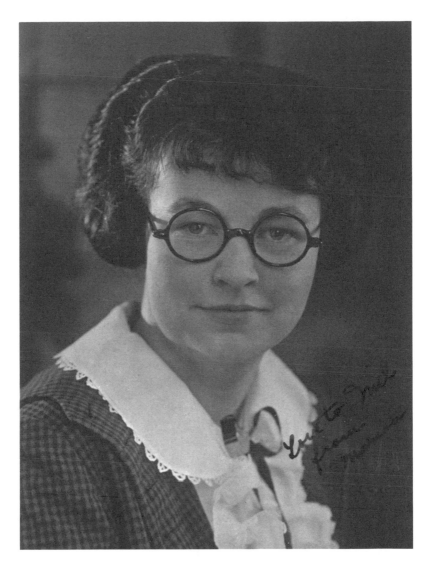

College graduation (1926)

I wasn't counting on this celebration to improve Mom's accuracy about her age. Instead her birthday was to be an occasion for her—and for us together—to celebrate and to enjoy. It was an event being observed. We were creating yet another island together in the ceaseless flow of time.

By reaching back into the uniqueness of their young-years together, she had given my mother what only a sister or brother could have given as a gift.

The Gift

"Look what came in the mail!" I said. She had greeted me as she always did, her face lighting up with a wonderful glow of pleasure and recognition. And then always a warm kiss on the cheek and sometimes a gentle caress of my face or hair. A wonderful reward for coming. But this time I also had a package for her.

"It's from your sister Mil." Her face lit up. "Mil knew it was your birthday, and she's sent you something," I said. I was starting to open the outer wrapping because I knew Mom couldn't get inside even an envelope these days, let alone a sealed package. The gift was wrapped in white tissue paper with a pink bow, which we admired. We were both caught up in the wonderful gift of anticipation that comes along with the gift itself.

"Mil has sent you some perfume!" I said. "Here, smell this." I had uncapped the cologne and, taking Mom's hand, I lightly sprayed her wrist.

"Ooh!" she exclaimed.

"Did that frighten you? Was that too cold on your wrist?" I asked. "Let me spray it on my hand and I'll put some on your other wrist."

I also put some on either side of her neck beneath her ears, as I had seen her do for herself so many times. She was very pleased.

Remembrances

"Does that fragrance remind you of anything?" I asked. "Did you ever smell that before?"

She was enjoying the aroma inwardly and smiling. My questions seemed beside the point or beyond her answering. At least she made no attempt to respond as she usually does. She was simply enjoying. She was self-absorbed in a wonderful inward reverie for twenty minutes or so, until I finally kissed her good-bye and left.

A subsequent letter from her sister, responding to my thank-you on my mother's behalf, told me what I had suspected. She had not chosen the fragrance casually. This was a fragrance that long ago my mother had selected for herself. Mil thought it went back to the time in 1923 or so when Mom and their older sister Ruth had been in Paris and, she wrote, "Perhaps it was then when they had gotten to know the Coty perfumes." Ruth had selected Rose as her fragrance, my mother this one, and for Mil still another. It was as if the sisters had color-coded themselves. Mil's gift evoked that old code they shared: "This was you, this was *us,* when we were young and long-ago."

Until this gift, Mil had not known how to reach out to her sister, my mother, in her Alzheimer's isolation and across the miles and years. But now, by reaching back into the uniqueness of their young-years together, she had given my mother as a gift what only a sibling such as Mil (or Ruth, now long dead) could have given. She had evoked some of the oldest of sisterly memories and ties, those of young women together and dressing for special occasions. Sixty years later in the 1980s, she had been able to transport my mother back to the flapper-styles of their young-adult years in the Roaring Twenties.

The Help We Give One Another in Our Recalling

When Mil's letter interpreting her gift came, I read it to my mother after I had put more fragrance on her wrists and by her ears. I was bringing the bottle from home every day. I had learned earlier not to leave something like that about in her room. Other patients, more mobile than she but just as forgetful, were free to move everywhere and upon occasion they moved whatever was moveable. For example, during one recent visit I found among the pictures on my mother's bureau an additional photo nicely framed but of a total stranger looking adoringly at her infant. Someone had wanted to share that photo with Mom, had done so—and then forgotten to retrieve it. Mom's special fragrance would best appear for her from home with me. It would be something we would share together (and *I* would have to remember to bring it).

A part of their isolation now is not just
the Alzheimer's disease. It is also
a product of their not having, as most of us
do most of the time in our younger years,
a community of people who share and call
forth our memories. Memories don't
just happen, they are evoked.

Writing about the fragrances had gotten Mil into remembering too. Her letter was all about her older sisters and their circles of friends, about their mother ("strict but fair"), and about Ruth and her struggles as the oldest to grow up faster than their mother had thought appropriate ("rouge and lipstick and smoking").

"Is that the way you remember it was then?" I asked. "Pretty much," Mom replied. I talked of old photographs I remembered from albums, moments snapped from their summers at Nausauket on the shores of Rhode Island's Narragansett Bay before and during World War I. The long bathing suits for women. The old cars. The big sun hats. The photographs of groups of summertime companions, girlhood chums many of whom would be lifelong friends. When my parents retired to Florida, these were some of the people who came winters to see them.

From my mother's responses I couldn't tell how much she was remembering, except that she was pleased. And the next day she wanted to tell me about Mil and a couple from California who had a daughter, and Ruth. It was clear there was more, but she could no longer hold all that in focus long enough to fill in for me the additional details I would have needed in order to understand. Unlike parts of her life that I had shared, I had no helping context of my own memories with which to fill in and help her. Because I could not remember with her here, she could not remember (or at least share) it all. *That* was something her sister Mil was able to do for her. But I could not, at least not for those earlier decades in my mother's life.

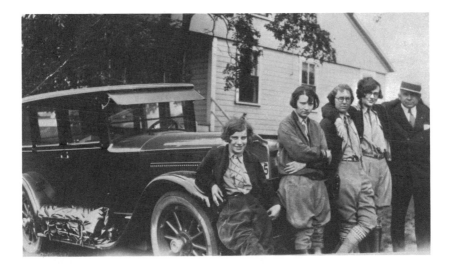

A camping trip over gravel roads from R.I. to Yellowstone National Park. (L to R) Mil, Ruth, Eleanor McLeod, Marion (or Pat) at 21 — and their father and driver Henry E. Fearney. (July 5, 1925)

I look at the other women and men in my mother's nursing home and I realize that a part of their isolation now is not just the Alzheimer's disease. It is also a product of their not having, as most of us do most of the time in our younger years, a community of people who share and call forth our memories. Memories don't just happen, they are evoked. Something brings them to mind. A fragrance. A birthday. A letter. A photograph. A visit. When for one reason or another you have largely moved beyond those who can share your memories, you become an emigrant, you have moved beyond and away from what used to be your home.

Celebrating in Order to Remember

The day we opened Mil's gift of fragrance a young nurse came in upon us as we were putting the perfume on. "It's my mother's birthday in just two days. She will be eighty-two," I said.

The young nurse beamed at my mother and burst into an animated rendition of "Happy Birthday To You," singing it all the way through to naming my mother by name, and then giving her a big congratulatory kiss on her cheek. My mother was thrilled.

"We were just putting on some of the perfume her sister Mil has sent."

"Yes," she said, "I can smell it. It's lovely, isn't it, Pat?" My mother glowed anew.

Several nights later, after my mother's birthday, I saw this young nurse again in the hallway and thanked her for her enthusiastic singing of the "Happy Birthday" song to my mother. "Your energy and spontaneity and enthusiasm are so wonderful," I told her, "they are such a special personal gift you have."

She told me that she had been on duty the next two days following my mother's birthday, and that every time she saw my mother or came into her room, she had given my mother that same rendition of "Happy Birthday." "She loved it every time," she said. I am sure my mother loved the attention, but I am also sure she loved being the one who evoked from this wonderful young person an expression of such youthful exuberance.

By the day after my mother's birthday, when I asked her if she had enjoyed it, she could say, "Yes," she had. Mil's gift of the fragrance, its repeated use, the memories it stirred, the many enthusiastic renditions of the Birthday Song, and my weaving a web orchestrating and connecting us all had allowed my mother access to a small community. We all joined her in celebrating her birthday in a way that neither she nor any of the rest of us, by ourselves, could have done. This time it had worked for her, for us.

I suddenly saw myself as a catalyst, one who by my presence could enable things to happen between my mother and other people that could not (or would not) happen "on their own."

I thought about how it happened. Mil's creative touching of my mother's sense of smell started it all. I also began to see that one of the functions I could play in my mother's life was as intermediary. By my thank-you note and report of Mom's response to her gift, I had unintentionally evoked a response from Mil in the form of Mil's memories. Through my aunt I had tapped into a whole stream of memories I did not share with my mother because I had not been born until later.

I realize also that I was functioning here in still another way. I used Mil's letter and Mil's memories to help my mother touch once again some times and places that, until then, had been long gone. I suddenly saw myself as a catalyst, one who by my presence could enable things to happen between my mother and other people that could not (or would not) happen "on their own."

All in all it had been quite a birthday. And now we were stepping off that small island, back into the rushing, flowing stream of time that washes through all our days.

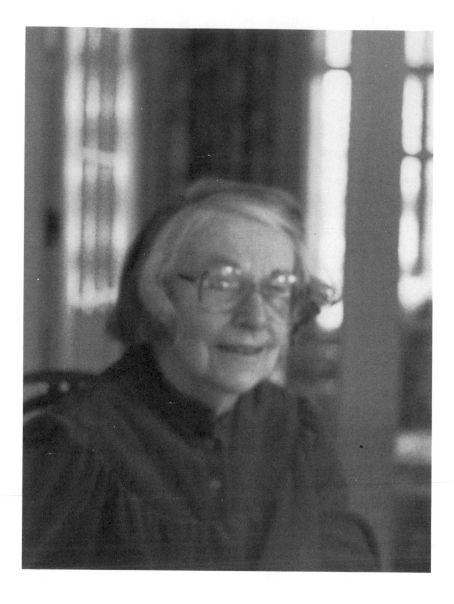

At home, Christmas 1983 (79½ years), seven months after diagnosis.

7.

Sunday Brightness

A Clearing in the Wood

I went over early to see my mother today, about 11:30. It is Sunday and a beautiful clear day. I am recently back from Dallas where I officiated at my niece's wedding. She is a lovely young woman of twenty-four and both she and her new husband have great personal energy and that elusive quality my wife and I call "sparkle" or personal charm and vitality. "It," I believe, is what Mom called it in her younger days.

Mom was bright, brighter than usual.
Her speech and her thinking were somewhat
garbled still but much better than most times, so we
had a simply wonderful time together.

My mother looked well. An energetic young nurse was combing her hair when I arrived. Several weeks to a month ago they had been having difficulty balancing off my mother's anti-blood-clotting medicine against her flesh bruising easily and her tearing her skin against things. That has all cleared up now, so her arms look a lot better. Most days she still wears the sort of anti-clotting stockings you have doubtless seen (or worn) in the hospital.

Mom was bright, brighter than usual. Her speech and her thinking were somewhat garbled still but much better than most times, so we had a simply wonderful time together. She spoke, for example, about "the day before yesterday"—a more complex description of time than I have heard from her since I can't remember when. At another point she interrupted her own thought and said, "My mother's dead, isn't she." It wasn't quite a statement, nor was it a complete question. But somehow today she could let herself know that her mother really was dead.

It was great good fortune that a card from her sister had come and also that I had it with me today. My first day back from Dallas I had not brought it; I saved my first visit for an account of the wedding and seeing my brother. She was so pleased with the card from her sister, first of all to get it. Then with the illustration. Then with the messages. Then (and this surprised me) with the envelope, where she looked for a long time at her sister's monogram embossed on the back of the envelope. She turned the envelope over and looked for a long time at her sister's handwriting, and then read aloud from our address on the envelope.

"Where," she then asked me, "are they living now?" I told her what she had once known, that her sister and husband were living in Richmond in a retirement community. "Oh yes," she said.

I showed her a clipping her sister had enclosed from their college alumnae magazine. Did she remember Mary Toner? "Oh yes," she said, and stared at her picture for a long time. I had the feeling my mother was much closer today to the boundary zone between where she has been recently (the last year) and her earlier and younger self. That is not supposed to be the way Alzheimer's works because with memory "once it's gone it's gone," or so I am told. Also I do not find my mother forgetting recent things any more than long-ago things. Both seem equally present but fuzzy. Distant past and recent past seem equally accessible to her when she is experiencing emotions that appropriately recall them.

"Give Liz My Love"

I told Mom for the first time that my wife Liz was home sleeping, napping; that she had been in the hospital again for surgery, this time on her other breast. Mom understood this perfectly and immediately asked, "How is she?" I told her (as I would tell you) that her surgeon and his pathologist colleague did not find any cancer cells but they did find a lot of cells that were not right—"hyperplasia," they called it. And the surgeon removed thirty percent of her breast. She was operated on this past Thursday, spent Thursday and Friday nights in the hospital and came home Saturday. She is sleeping a lot and watching the US Tennis Open on television with the help of our VCR. Last night before we went to bed, she put on a sweater and wrap and we went down a flight of stairs, out our front door, and walked around our two nearest courtyards for fifteen minutes before it was enough. (We usually walk for an hour or more each night before we go to bed).

> My mother has a much greater grasp of
> the meaning and significance of what I convey
> to her than oftentimes her garbled responses
> allow her to express.

But what bothers Liz is the sense of being nibbled away at, and the pain-pain-PAIN of a post-mastectomy frozen shoulder. She is barely well after thirty-four months and she has had two more operations to remove portions of her remaining breast. She has the sense that her body is continuing to produce stuff that pathologists regard as precancerous. All this is not the sort of thing to encourage Liz about her current well-being or prospective longevity.

I did not go into all the detail with Mom, but into much of it. We went on to talk of other things. I then told her I was going to leave,

I had to go to the supermarket and get some groceries and make Liz her lunch. I kissed Mom good-bye and told her I would see her tomorrow. As I turned to leave, she called me back and then said very clearly, "Give Liz my love."

That is not standard or boilerplate conversation between us. I take that as evidence my mother has a much greater grasp of the meaning and significance of what I convey to her than oftentimes her garbled responses allow her to express. What she did today was to give me a completely appropriate farewell for the conversation she remembered we had been having about five minutes earlier!

It is a moment of insight in which I-the-man suddenly confront the boy both in myself and in the photograph. I-the-man am now remembering how it was when that moment was being snatched from time onto a bit of photographic paper. I realize that being with my mother in her Alzheimer's disease has stimulated in me my own need to remember, and also my interest in pondering this amazing process of recollection, of memory.

Peering Backward into Time through Old Photos

One of the things that came from seeing my brother and his wife was that Rick dug out his collection of old family photographs. One was a 1909 photo (next page) of our mother and her older-by-one-year sister Ruth as First Graders at the Shaw Avenue Elementary School in Edgewood, R.I. My mother is third from the left in the front row; her sister Ruth is second from the right. There were also photographs of my father's mother's family, the Sperrys. I know

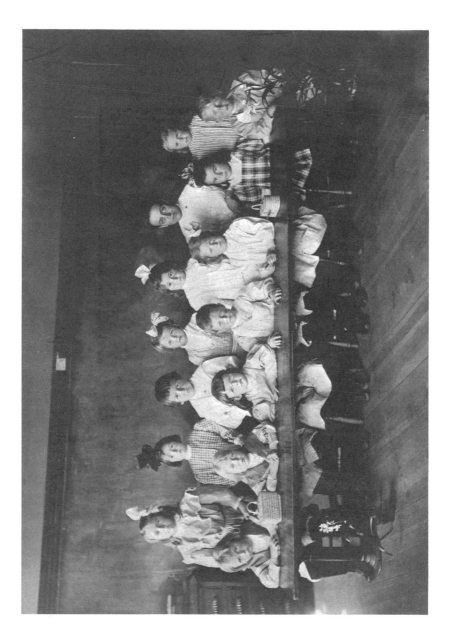

of these people by name and by family tombstone but they died before I was born and I had never seen them in pictures.

My brother's old family photographs handed down from my mother were quite different from those I had received from her. I found I wanted my own copies of all these moments snatched by a photographer and a camera from our family's onward rush of being alive. One was a photograph of a family group, taken when our mother was even younger. I wanted to know who the rest of those people were. Would my aunt in Richmond, though born later, recognize them or this place?

I can recall still today the moment in which one photograph (next page) of a family gathering was being taken. It was at the Vernon Stiles Inn in Thompson, Connecticut, in the summer of 1937. My mother's cousin Karl was the photographer. He was 43 then and I was fascinated that his camera had a timer so he could step from behind the camera lens and into the photograph. And there I am in the photograph, a boy of seven, watching all this and being photographed. And remembering. That was more than half a lifetime ago for Karl; for me it is a moment of mysterious insight in which I-the-man suddenly confront the boy both in myself and in the photograph. I-the-man am now remembering how it was when that moment was being snatched from time onto a bit of photographic paper. I realize that being with my mother in her Alzheimer's disease has stimulated in me my own need to remember, and also my interest in pondering this amazing process of recollection, of memory, by which the past is so wonderfully retrieved and, as astronomers do for distant stars with a radio telescope, a past moment is brought into the present.

Standing in the Middle of the Stream

It is also absolutely clear from these old family photographs that my brother's forehead and hairline come from our father's grand-father Jared Sperry—and mine do not. My forehead looks more

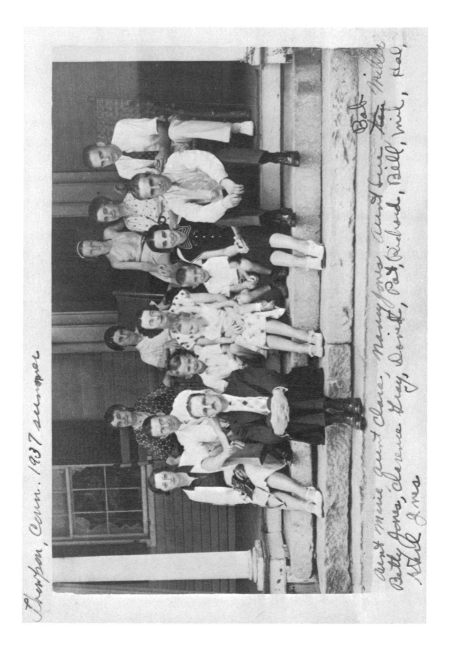

Thompson, Conn. 1937 summer

Aunt Marie, Aunt Clara, Mary Jane, Aunt Lion, Tom, Miller, Bob
Betty Jones, Clarence Gray, Dorott, Pat, Richard, Bill, mil, Hal,
Etal, Irma

like that of our mother's grandfather Charles Parisette, whose image I have seen in a photograph of him in his Civil War beard, medal and uniform. My appearance, like his and his grandson Karl's, is one of thinning hair, receding forehead, and increasingly craggy features. I wish we had photographs of my father's other grandparents. My father seems clearly not to have taken after his father but to have looked more like Jared Sperry, his maternal grandfather, as does my brother.

I showed my mother these family portraits and talked with her about my reactions to them. She nodded with interest and, I thought, with recognition. I realize my own reactions to the photographs comes from my currently acute awareness of standing in the middle between generations. The younger generation of our children is old enough and sufficiently formed for us to be in wonder at their youth and aspirations. How like themselves they are—and yet like us, and like our parents and grandparents and so on. The stream of life flows ever on in us, through us, over us. Like rocks in a mountain stream we are gradually shaped and worn down by so much living, until that living is gone.

8.

Last Love-Song

Gone But Not-Gone?

Is this the way it all ends? I asked myself. My mother today seems much quieter, much more still, much less vital. She is instead expressionless and emotionally withdrawn. Since she is not talking, I talk.

My mother seems to be fading out, "like a distant radio station."

I often make conversation by telling her about my day, about the family, about phone calls she would be interested in hearing about. Usually she has reactions and soon interrupts me so that it is the two of us talking, and we talk together, even though neither one of us is understanding all of what the other is saying.

But this is different now.

My mother seems to be fading out, "like a distant radio station," I told someone. It is as though you are driving further and further away, and the signal is getting fainter and fainter. You know that soon you are going to go over some hill and lose the station altogether. But you drive up the next hill and regain the signal for a time. And you know you will then lose it again, and perhaps again. And then, you know, finally it will be gone for good.

Is that the way it is going to be? Long before she stops breathing, will she be gone? I see what I take to be patients in more advanced stages of Alzheimer's disease. They lie back in special chairs that support them half-sitting and half-lying while they sleep open-mouthed with knees drawn up like a sleeping child, sleeping away their last months and days and weeks, waking only to eat and be bathed and changed and dressed and, at evening, put back to bed.

I observe the gentle care the staff gives these more advanced Alzheimer's patients. I am grateful on their behalf, so to speak. But somehow I have never allowed myself to think of my mother becoming like them. That is still difficult for me to think about and feel. I have wondered, too, about the apparent policy of having patients who are sleeping away their days staying still in the common room, surrounded by those also with Alzheimer's who are so much better off.

Can We Really See What's Coming?

Won't it be depressing for those who are better off to see those who now sleep—to see those who are closer to death but have not died yet?

I suddenly realize I feel squeamish about being so blunt. I feel like a Victorian, someone from that earlier era when there were some things which, it was thought, are best not discussed. It was as though by not naming these parts of our human experience, their status as social realities would be effectively denied. But dying, like sex, is there for all of us regardless. It is just that most of us have to come to grips with sex and death at such utterly different points in our life span.

I find myself imagining the unit administrator's point of view: on which particular day is one to decide that XYZ will no longer come to the common room with everyone else? So unless the patients protest, they continue to be present for the shared life of the unit—even if they sleep through most of it. If their dozing is light, it provides for them a familiar daily cycle of music and meals and activities. On the other hand if their dozing is deep, it all does not matter. Who among us really knows how much around them those deeply dozing patients follow? Who knows what thoughts or dreams come to their minds?

It is the advocates of the disabled who remind us that we are the temporarily able-bodied, and that for many of us our time of illness or disability will come, sometime.

But what of the other patients who are better off? What do they make of their dozing neighbors?

They seem to be taking it all in stride, much as you and I do when we are walking down the street somewhere. If we encounter someone on crutches or someone piloting a motorized wheelchair, we accept their being there as a part of our urban landscape: we do not expect to be all alike. It is the advocates of the disabled who remind us that we are the temporarily able-bodied, and that for many of us our time of illness or disability will come, sometime.

There is actually a remarkably acute perception of one another among the patients in my mother's Alzheimer's unit. I have gradually become aware that my mother really knows this one, and then that one, and then another. She knows them in the way you or I know people we see regularly in church or in a large office or at a club. She knows them in a neighborly way: they are not strangers to her, she has contact with them, she speaks to them and they to her (though it is mostly in garble).

One night my mother, while I was helping her eat supper, interrupted my helping her with the next mouthful. "Are you having tears?" she asked aloud very clearly, and I knew she was not speaking to me. I turned to see who she was speaking to. "Hello, Clara," I said, "I'm sorry I have been sitting with my back to you while I have been talking with my mother." "You're sad," my mother said to Clara. And Clara continued to look at my mother very sadly.

My mother's perception of Clara's depressed emotional state seemed to me right on target. And it seemed clear to me that my mother was concerned for her friend, her neighbor, though my mother was severely limited in the help she could be to Clara. It also seemed to me evident that my mother could speak her thoughts most clearly about what was emotionally so vivid to her, her neighbor's continuing sadness.

If this is my mother's perception not only of Clara but of Frances and Sarah and Ed and Wilma and Sadie and Doris and Sophie and Rosie and Bill and the rest, then I suppose she also sees and makes something of the other Ed who most days dozes in his special chair all day, waking only for meals. I do not know whether my mother realizes that now she too spends her days not in an ordinary wheelchair but in one of those special chairs. It is flexible and adjustable and much more comfortable for her. But does she see it as a part of her progression toward a life of dozing, like the other Ed? I don't know what she may see or feel about this; she does not say, or if she does, I have not understood it.

Grieving Being Apart

We had been away for nearly three weeks. First each of us were on business trips, and then, while we were on the West Coast, we stayed and saw our daughter for eight days in San Diego. I talked with my mother about our travel for a week or more before we left.

By the time we left, she was remembering we were going. The last few days she was surprised by my visits. "I thought you had left," she would say to me each night quite lucidly. "No, not yet," I would say, and finally it came to "No, we leave tomorrow, Liz for Washington State and I for Connecticut."

When I reappeared after eighteen days away, I found my mother very emotionally withdrawn. Had she had gone downhill *because* I had been away? I told myself that I was but a small fraction of her daily experience, thirty minutes or an hour at the most each day.

Or was it that I had been so close to her, seeing her every day, and it took a trip and the time apart in order for me to perceive suddenly how there was no longer a match between my mental remembrance of her and her actual condition? I have seen this phenomenon in myself when our children were young: they seemed to have grown so much even when I had been gone from them only for a week. I concluded this was not possible; it must be that day by day I was not seeing them clearly and only updated my perception of them periodically. Was I updating my perception of my mother now in that same sort of way?

When I reappeared after eighteen days away, I found my mother very emotionally withdrawn. Was it that she had gone downhill *because* I had been away?

All this was rushing through my mind. Self-blame. Worry about my mother. Concern about her future. And concern about my future with her. Is this the way our relationship ends? Is it going to be like a sidewalk drawing in colored pastel chalk that just becomes more and more blurred, until the picture is erased and gone?

Finding New Strategies

Walking home after seeing my mother I realized this was a new concern for me. I had not been allowing myself to think about what was coming. I concentrated instead on living each day with my mother as much as we could. I still think that's a good strategy. But suddenly I was *having* to think ahead, as I tried to understand what I was seeing now, and what was happening that was new.

The next week or so I spent more time just listening when I visited my mother, just being with her and, as always, holding her hand. Gradually she wanted to talk more. I kept listening, kept encouraging. I had stopped telling her much at all about our lives outside her immediate and present world. I concentrated on going even further into her garble and her world. There were many days I did not grasp even three or four words that suggested a coherent line of thought. The words were pouring out of my mother again, but their meaning wasn't coming along with them.

The words were pouring out of my mother again, but their meaning wasn't coming along with them.

Sometimes they were like the words of someone reading a dictionary. Sometimes they were sequences of numbers, such as four-three-seven-two. Occasionally there were names. Finally one day my mother tried to tell me about walking up a path to a house at the top of a hill and the house was painted with red. Her description, though elaborate for her nowadays, did not trigger any memory I could recall sharing with her. But it was clear that Mom knew quite precisely the place she wanted to be telling me about.

I felt encouraged.

I began to think that Mom had been experiencing (and I had become involved in her experiencing) a period in which she had really become quite depressed. That would account for her seeming so emotionally withdrawn and expressionless. But it was clear that she was coming out of it now, and hence I was feeling encouraged.

It may have been a shift in her medications; that would account for such a change. It might be simply a change in how her body was reacting to the medications she had been getting all along. Or most likely of all, Mom may have been going through a period in which she was emotionally in touch with her own grieving, her own mourning the passing of her last days.

It may be that one of the functions for her of my daily visits is to re-attach her to what she has accomplished in this life, what she has felt good about. My visits do mean to her (and to me) the reassertion of caring and companionship and meaning amid increasingly difficult limits. Our trip to the West Coast, our absence of eighteen days, may have withdrawn that reassurance and allowed my mother to get in touch with her sadness about all her limitations now and about all that is passing and has passed out of her life.

My mother's perception of Clara's sadness suggests to me that my mother knows sadness can go with these days and circumstances. With or without Alzheimer's, such sadness is a part of everyone's drawing near to their own dying. The only alternative is that, like the spaceship Challenger's sudden and disastrous demise, it happens in a twinkling, a catastrophic moment. And then we who are left are apt to mourn that abrupt departure as premature. "Premature" or "prolonged," we do not like dying either way.

"Lullaby, and Goodnight"

One night shortly after our return and before my mother had become more reengaged with her world and with me, I arrived a little later than usual. She had just had her shower and she was clearly on her way to bed.

She was sitting up brightly in the nurses' station, dressed in a clean hospital johnny and seated on a simply wheeled chair. Around her were other patients, some ambulatory, others awaiting their baths or showers as they sat in their wheelchairs. Amid the chatter of conversation presided over by George, a young male aide, my mother's hair was being dried with an electric blow-drier and brush. Mom sat on the wheeled chair as though on a throne, for she was at the center of everyone's attention. She reminded me of a child getting one of their first haircuts at a barbershop: she was a little apprehensive but also pleased with all the attention.

When her hair was dried, George told me to wait just a minute while he got my mother into her bed. He came out shortly and I went in to sit with her for a few minutes. He had left the lights on for me, and since they were clearly in Mom's eyes, I dimmed them to the night-light level.

We sat there in the semi-darkness, I holding her hand and she now staring at the ceiling, still emotionally distant and withdrawn. I was intruding upon her bedtime, I realized; I must not stay too long and interfere with her going to sleep. It was about 7:20 P.M. and sometimes, I knew, she was asleep by 7:00.

It was not a time for me to talk, and she seemed done with talking herself for the day. Then I suddenly connected with all the times I sat with our children while they were going to sleep. I couldn't rub my mother's back as I had rubbed theirs, for she was lying on her back. But I told Mom about how Liz and I sang our children lullabies. Then I started singing softly to my mother all the lullabies I could remember from some twenty to twenty-eight years earlier.

I don't think my mother ever sang lullabies to my brother or me. I don't think I ever heard my mother sing except hymns in church. And when she helped me memorize "McNamara's Band" when I was eight or nine. But that night I sang eight or ten or perhaps a dozen lullabies and love-songs we had wooed our children with. Walking home afterward I wondered what my mother made of those fifteen or twenty minutes together.

I will never know. But I was doing for my mother what Liz and I did for our children, and it felt very good to be able to parent my mother in a way different from, but like, the ways she had loved and parented me.

9.

Seeing Sophie

Visits from Long-Dead Relatives

I think I have finally found the key to understanding something that has puzzled me. When I come late in the day to sit with my mother for half an hour or so, she frequently talks in her Alzheimer garble about seeing "Muthie" (the way she always pronounced the word *mother* when speaking of her own mother) and also about seeing Ruth, her long-dead sister.

They were always close, living not in each other's shadow but in each other's sunlight.

I always affirm these reports, asking her such things as how they were, or did they have much to say, or other things I have learned may evoke further comments or explanations from her.

It was always a great satisfaction to my mother to report these visits, as she was very close to them both. As a boy our family had lived not half a mile from my mother's childhood home where her parents still lived. Her mother was very much a part of my own mother's adult life as well as of mine. When my grandmother finally became ill with cancer, my mother nursed her in our home during those final weeks and her mother died in my mother's arms. Yes, they were close.

She was very close to Ruth too. Ruth was little more than a year ahead of my mother, and their mother entered them in school the same year, as though they were twins. When they went on to high school, each had their own circle of friends and activities. I have been told that by my other aunt, and I have seen it in the accounts of senior year written for their senior yearbook. They were always close, living not in each other's shadow but in each other's sunlight. Ruth died of cancer in her early fifties, now more than thirty years ago.

But all this family history of women's friendships did not account for my mother's reports of seeing Muthie and Ruth now. Like reports of UFO sightings, I was inwardly disbelieving. I was certain there must be some other explanation, and I bided my time.

Delusions, or Fantasies?

Despite the losses attributable to my mother's Alzheimer's disease, I function with my mother on the assumption that whatever my mother is telling me, though garbled, is still rational, still coherent, still a reflection of the same reality we have always known and loved and shared together. Perhaps the image of reality now is not smooth and continuous like a photographic image. It is more like an image seen in a stained-glass window which is laced with lead, breaking the image into many little pieces. The important thing for my mother and for me is that it still is, to both of us, a recognizable image of our once-upon-a-time world together.

But sightings (or "visits") from her mother and Ruth challenged all this. It made me wonder if I was now crossing over into my mother's dream-world. I remember the first symptom which had alerted any of us (including my mother) to Alzheimer's disease, which was her reporting to Karl at breakfast that she had seen some worms crawling on the step to her bathroom in his home.

Seeing the worms had triggered an entire sequence of events. It was like the sudden and multiple moves that my grandmother had been so good at when I played childhood checkers, an entire sequence of moves that suddenly ended the game. My mother had gone quickly from their internist to a psychiatrist to a neuropsychiatrist to hospital tests, and then her nearly lifelong excellent health was, like the checkers game, suddenly at an end. At eighty or eighty-one she "had Alzheimer's."

We continued to enjoy her at home with Karl for a year or two. She forgot words more and more frequently. Our conversations on the phone increasingly became monologues in which she was listening to us tell her about our lives and our children's lives. She still enjoyed this a great deal, but she was no longer as able to take her earlier share of the initiative in a conversation.

But during all this time I never sensed that my mother's reality was becoming vastly different from our own. There was a difficult period, unrelated to her Alzheimer's, when she was hospitalized for a week for tests—and she became very disoriented. But when she returned to her familiar place and routines and people she sprang back to where she had been before hospitalization.

Her reporting of reality was becoming more and more garbled now, and I came to see that her perception of what we were saying was getting garbled as well. Her visits from Muthie and Ruth were starkly different. Had she dreamt these?

Dreams and Dream-Visits?

We all dream. But most of what we dream we don't remember. Or we soon forget it. We also daydream, which is different. Daydreams are the thoughts which float into our consciousness "out of nowhere," apparently unstimulated by the external reality that is passing before our eyes, unstimulated even by the conscious mental reality we would say we are "thinking about." Daydreams are the stuff Sigmund Freud noticed. In creating psychoanalysis, he used these daydreams along with our sleeping dreams as clues to otherwise invisible and unperceived contents of our emotional life. This is all very helpful in gaining access to important but hidden psychological structures when there is need or desire to amend them, change them. When I was getting my graduate theological training more than three decades ago, I spent three and a half intensive years in psychoanalysis. I knew (and know) something about how to move with dreams or daydreams, how to float in a stream of consciousness and learn from its flow and eddies.

My mother's reports of seeing her mother and sister did not seem to me like reports of either sleeping dreams or daydreams. I see no reason (yet) to think Alzheimer patients do not dream nightdreams when they sleep. Like all the rest of us they too seem able to have dreams of those long dead. Likewise those who are now long-dead can suddenly pop into consciousness and seemingly materialize into our mind's eye and our present flow of conscious thoughts that "just come to mind."

But what my mother was saying seemed different from someone talking about what had merely come to mind in a dream while asleep or as a passing thought. What my mother was talking about clearly seemed to her to be an actual event that she was reporting, something as firm and as matter-of-fact as anything that someone with Alzheimer's disease ever talks about.

What, I wondered, is going on?

A Look-Alike and Sound-Alike

My sense of there being still a shared reality between my mother and me was strengthened many months earlier when I discovered a look-alike and sound-alike in the nursing home for her cousin Karl. I was with her when my mother heard Ed Fitzgerald's voice and called out to him by her cousin Karl's name.

Both men are large-boned, tall, well-built with some handsomeness and distinction. Both are now more frail with age, but their voices still speak with precision and authority. The great difference of course is that Ed is a fellow patient; Ed has Alzheimer's and my mother sees him every day, while Karl was my mother's lifelong favorite older cousin. After the death of my father and of Karl's wife, Karl had needed someone to run his home, and my mother returned from Florida to live with Karl for nearly a decade.

Alzheimer's, I realized, was diminishing my mother's capacity for precise perceptions as well as for precise expression of ideas. So her confusing Ed with Karl made sense. While they are not precise look-alikes or sound-alikes, there are similarities which she had noted and was responding to. Over the months I have seen her continue responding to Ed's voice and his movements around the common room. I also know that most of the time my mother knows that Ed is not Karl and that Karl is at home in Barrington—and that I bring her news of Karl from time to time as I see or talk with him.

But would I find other such clues to my mother's apparent confusions?

While they are not precise look-alikes or sound-alikes, there are similarities which she had noted and was responding to.

My Discovery of a Key

I said earlier, I think I finally discovered a possible clue to the minor mystery of my mother's visits from her dead mother and sister. It happened while we were in the common room. My mother was, with my help, eating her supper. The room was as usual full of patients eating. Some were eating by themselves, others were being helped by staff, some had eaten at an earlier sitting and were strolling about.

One who was walking after dinner was someone I had come to know slightly, Sophie. She is perhaps 5'-4", slightly shorter than my mother in her prime. Sophie is still a vigorous walker. But this night Sophie came up close to where my mother and I were. We were seated just in front of a lovely gilt-frame wall mirror, and Sophie kept coming back to behold her own image in it. She would stare for fifteen or twenty seconds, walk away, and then in a minute or two come back.

I have always spoken to Sophie, greeting her as I came in. As a minister I long ago acquired the habit of noticing people's names and then thereafter greeting them by name. But the second or third time Sophie came and stood by my mother and peered into the mirror, I said to my mother, "You know Sophie, don't you?" Sophie turned for a moment from the mirror, peered at me and at my mother, and then returned to the mirror. My mother garbled something—and suddenly I connected.

I said to my mother—or to Sophie (I forget, because I was excited): "Her name is the same as your mother's name. She's another Sophie, isn't she!"

"Sophie"—An Unusual Name My Mother Kept Hearing

I knew the staff talked a lot to Sophie because she was mobile. Sophie was also widely known in the unit as a mooch; she was always fed at the first sitting and, if she were still hungry, she would go like a pirate from table to table liberating for herself whatever she liked from other patients' trays, especially those patients too slow or too unable to protect their own suppers.

Even after Sophie had finished her own supper, she would sidle up to a table silently and snatch a dessert-cookie or a portion of cake with frosting. It was clear she had a lifelong sweet tooth, and she was not used to just one dessert.

All this meant that "Sophie" was a name frequently heard in the common room. The staff, among their other duties, had to keep an eye out or an ear cocked for Sophie. Like a smiling two and a half year old, she was loveable but you had to watch her.

I now think that my mother, hearing her mother's name so frequently, felt that her mother was nearby, there, somewhere, within calling distance—and she told me about it. I have not checked yet to find if there is also a patient (or staff person) with her sister Ruth's name. But it would not surprise me now to find a "Ruth."

All of us have similar experiences on the street: we see someone whose face or build or gait or laugh remind us of someone we know. Why then should we expect to give that up when we get old or have Alzheimer's disease?

Further Confirmation

As I was leaving that night I met Sophie's son arriving to see his mother. I told him of my discovery. He laughed, for he knows his mother well. He then told me of their family's similar experience. Sophie was talking to him for some time about seeing Goldie, her now-deceased sister. "Goldie's been here," she would tell him, much as my mother spoke of her mother and Ruth.

Sophie's son told me it was his sister who had recognized that another patient had the tight Blondie-like curls, the fair skin, and a general similarity of build to Sophie's sister Goldie. Another look-alike.

When I got home, my wife's reaction was that all of us have similar experiences on the street: we see someone whose face or build or gait or laugh remind us of someone we know. Why then should we expect to give that up when we get old or have

Alzheimer's disease? That's how we have always recognized one another, by patterns that look and sound familiar.

I feel even more sure now about my mother's sanity amid all her garbled Alzheimer's talk. A few weeks before I "saw Sophie," you'll recall I was visiting my mother on a day when her head was especially clear and she said to me, apropos of absolutely nothing, "Muthie's dead, isn't she." At her best moments my mother is still sorting out these realities. And doing it accurately, at least at her best.

I am grateful I persisted in my conviction that my mother's reality is still continuous with her own (and my) old shared reality. I am grateful I kept listening seriously most of the time. And I am grateful that, this once at least, my persistence was rewarded with a key to one mystery.

It is important to me to continue to live with my mother in a shared reality and not to feel that—because of her Alzheimer's disease—she has passed over into some alien and totally strange land in which her life experiences no longer make sense to her or to anyone else.

10.

Old Sunlight

I came upon a memory the other day
in a most unexpected way.
It was a piece of fabric, green-plaid with purple,
from a shirt of long ago.
No more than four-by-four, it opened a window
into a long-gone past
and suddenly old sunlight was shining
in the midst of my today.

That long-gone shirt was a favorite, of course.
Details are gone now but it had been a present from my mother
when I was a teenage boy and she a mid-years woman,
oh nearly forty years ago.
It was a shirt she had made up herself
on her sewing machine,
working in the sun on the shiny mahogany expanse
of our dining room table.

I can remember my fascination with the processes,
the laying colored-side against colored-side
and getting the plaids matched
so "left" would look like "right."
I can remember holding the tension on the fabric
so she could cut, cut, cut

with the special scissors.
Where are those scissors now?

How her shiny little Singer machine
would whir and whir and whir,
pulsing thread and shape and life into fabric,
holding it tight
until it became the shape and design and garment
in which we lived.

I did not know then that life is like that.
Perhaps I thought life happened
or at best you did some things to it.
What I did not grasp until later was how each day
we are putting the pieces together
into which we live the real life we live.
Dreams mattered then, and consequences were still unreal.

But today I saw pieces of that long-ago still with us,
a seamless garment of selfhood
closer than breath or skin.
We are accustomed to the darkness surrounding
all we don't see or can no longer usually hold in mind.
But in that piece of remembered fabric,
found now after so long,
suddenly I discovered a magic mirror to peer in.
For a moment I could glimpse and experience
a boy I no longer am.
I could feel the brilliance of old sunlight
pouring into a long ago window
in a moment more poignant now
than my mother or I could ever have dreamt of then,
so long now ago.

11.

Looking for a Map

I find that I am thinking these days a great deal about aging. About my own growing older and about my mother's growing older. What I need, I know, is some sort of intellectual map, a way of locating myself not in space but in time. This is certainly not something our shared cultural experience provides us.

Not only do we lack adequate intellectual maps of
the time ahead in our personal life spans that we are
moving into, but I have concluded that
there literally is no road ahead
and we are making it as we go.

Perhaps our lack of such maps with which to orient ourselves is due to our experiencing such rapid social change. We are all moving into a society which has never existed before. The old, like the young, are (as Margaret Mead observed) immigrants in time. We not only lack maps but in many respects we lack the necessary experience. For example, I have never been this age until now, and in many respects it has been a different year in my life than last year when I was a year younger. Likewise, my mother has never had Alzheimer's disease before. Not only do we lack adequate intellectual maps of the time ahead in our personal life spans that we are moving into, but I have concluded that there literally is no road ahead and we are making it as we go.

I come back to what have purported to be the equivalent of maps, and what too often we take to be maps and then try to orient our lives by. We must look at these.

"The Hill of Life"

When we were youngsters in elementary school or slightly older, I think we accepted without questioning that each year was supposed to mean a "higher" grade. It was a mountain-climbing image or "We are climbing Jacob's ladder." Our parents talked about "when you grow *up.*"

In this way of thinking, "growing old" or "aging" is simply the other side of the hill of life.

A corollary of this was adulthood, which was talked about as "the prime of life." Adulthood in this mythology was a prolonged peak experience—"being a grownup." I think all of us who made it to being adults are agreed that adulthood has been for each of us many different things, but certainly the comprehensive term we would use to describe all of adulthood would not be "peak experience."

In this way of thinking, "growing old" or "aging" is simply the other side of the hill of life. We stroll down into retirement and senility and dying. Some seem to stumble down that side of the hill of life, others actually plummet. But whatever the mode of the aging, it was thought of as down, down, down.

From my perspective in the life span, such a mental map is not useful. It is not adequate to what I see happening, and it is clearly a map drawn by or for children who have not been my age—or my mother's age—yet. With luck they will live so long. Then they too will find they need a different map.

"Life Is Growth, To Be Alive Is Always To Be Growing"

Another map of life I find many people in their forties using depicts life as "growth." The original sin according to this life map is not always to be growing. Or—heaven forbid—to regress, to go back to an earlier stage of maturity or immaturity.

On this map personal growth is usually sketched for us in very male terms, so that the events which provide milestones for our "growing up" are perceived as involving letting go. Life is seen as a long string of lettings-go of someone or someplace and striking out on a path or journey to something new and "more fulfilling," meaning more self-sufficient and more "free." "Free" in this context often is an empty notion, without specific content but assumed to be an important and positive value. Nowhere on this map is it spelled out what we are free to become or free to be, except we are free "to be ourselves."

The Growth Map encourages me to look back and see I began this life-long process of separating when I let go of Mother's apron strings and first went to school. Life is a succession of such lettings-go. I let go of my first teacher and the security of that familiarity, to go on to my next grade. I let go of home each time we moved. Adulthood in this scenario means "getting your license" (so you can be free enough and "grown enough" to drive by yourself). Or it means joining the Army and "becoming a man." For girls it used to mean getting married. But despite women talking about "growing," it seems to me that by this life-map the traditional girl, when she becomes the traditional woman, ceases needing to grow up. She moves from her father's care and responsibility to her husband's care and responsibility. Growing up and becoming her own woman is something she stumbles into later when she divorces, or when the children grow up and she is without her built-in at-home job. For some women it happens when they are widowed.

On the Growth Map, adulthood is the end-result of all these separations: you are independent from your parents, you stand on your own two feet. Many a man in his mid-life crisis resumes this pattern of growth-by-separation. He leaves his wife of fifteen or twenty years with the rationale that his life is stifling him, he needs space, he needs to grow. So he leaves, and presumably he grows. At the least he is free of that wife and free to take another.

If "growth" means self-sufficiency and being free to run your own life, then the Growth Map describes it. But this map does not show anyone how relationships are started or how these relationships are nurtured over a lifetime. Nor does this map give any clues as to how we weather storms and hard times and illnesses with the help of one another. Nor does it lead us to expect that we might bring to our older years more resources in personal relationships than we started out with when we were first married, or first established a professional or personal friendship, or first knew the various members of our family of origin.

Intellectual maps must certainly account for our individuating into centers of initiative and desire and creativity and accountability. But an adequate map must also give adequate renderings of how, as we go along in life, we can learn to manage increasingly complex networks of commitments, caring and relationships. More and more it seems to me that these invisible connections are the stuff from which meaning and nurturance in our later years are built.

Adulthood As An Extended Plateau

What I see happening with my mother and many of our other dear older friends is that their later years have much in common with a vast plain or an extended plateau that goes on and on. This is not to deny that energies fade earlier in the day as we grow older. But we also can learn to recharge ourselves with naps.

To speak of aging as an extended plateau is *not* to join those elders among us who still want to claim that really *they* are "growing younger" each year. What they seem usually to mean by such silliness is that *they* are not on any slippery slope called "aging." When what they mean is that they arc not over the hill, I can agree with that. But like wine they too are aging day by day.

What it seems to me can be said is that, as we grow older, often there is a trade-off between wisdom and energy. This is summed up in a maxim some friends have on the door of their refrigerator, to the effect that "Old age and treachery will overcome youth and ambition." After we have absorbed the guffaw provoked by this maxim, we can recognize in it both the confidence and the wisdom of the older person, as well as the superior energy and often the idealism and visionary powers of the younger person.

Nor is life a game of solitaire in which one plays primarily against oneself, trying to uncover and "play" as many "cards" as there are hidden in one's pile of days.

We do change as we age. We changed as we went from infancy to childhood to adolescence to adulthood too. To live is to change, and aging is simply another part of that continuing lifelong process.

Yes, there are some losses as we age and change. There are also some gains. Life is not simply a bridge game in which one is to play out one's "cards" and "try to take as many tricks" as one can. Nor is life a game of solitaire in which one plays primarily against oneself, trying to uncover and "play" as many "cards" as there are hidden in one's pile of days.

I think that as we age increasing numbers of us are realizing that "winning" in this life may not even involve staying in the game until every possible card in the deck is played. An adequate intellectual map of a life span, it seems to me, involves leaving early enough and promptly, without stringing out the good-byes or spoiling the end of the evening by wishing that it (or we) were still young.

Having said that energies ebb, and earlier said that depths of relationships may be ripening in many directions and dimensions of our lives as we age, then I have to take account of why Old Age has gotten such a bad press among the young.

I think Old Age or growing old is often confused by us with the many disastrous and instantaneous transformations of life to which the human condition has been prone from the first moment of our conception. Futures planners have a word for these events; they call them "discontinuities." The Fall of the Roman Empire was such a discontinuity in Western culture, and it ushered in more than five hundred years of what we have called the Dark Ages.

Old Age or growing old is often confused by us with the many disastrous and instantaneous transformations of life to which the human condition has been prone from the first moment of our conception.

It is true that either at or on our way to our dying and our departing, everyone finally experiences such a transformation. This is what those who are younger observe and then confuse with Old Age or aging. Those in their thirties and forties observe that those older than they—precisely how much older moves along with you as you yourself age—do indeed have a disproportionate share of such instantaneous transformations.

For a long-time couple, the death of one's partner is one such catastrophic discontinuity. Suddenly everything is no longer as it was, and by this death and this severing of a vital relationship, one is indeed bereft and diminished. But this is not the only way it happens, and it is not only in our later years that this occurs.

"Instantaneous Transformations"

We know a person (usually a man) can suddenly drop dead of a heart attack in their fifties or sixties. It also happens to younger people, men (and also women) in their mid- and late thirties and, of course, in their forties. But we forget these early deaths remarkably fast. When we are in our thirties and forties, we do not think it is going to happen to us. After all we are *young,* and we are deeply into denying that possibility. The prime of life is not supposed to involve (for us) such instantaneous disasters and transformations. But it does, and heart disease is not the only example.

There are the AIDS patients. There are the auto accidents or skiing accidents from which a man (or a woman) emerges as a paraplegic (unable to walk and confined for the duration to a wheelchair-mobile existence) or a quadriplegic (paralyzed from the neck down and unable to use hands or legs). There are fatal mountain climbing accidents. In my mother's youth and in my own, poliomyelitis was prominent among the instantaneous transformations; my mother was stricken with polio while on a trip through Europe during the summer of her sophomore year in college. She lost a year of college and was fortunate, after being paralyzed in her right (or was it left) arm and leg, that both completely recovered except for their tendency to tire more quickly than the unaffected limbs.

We all know that the list of such instantaneous transformations is long. It extends now to the prenatal condition and to genetic (inherited) conditions. There have always been ways, a multitude of ways, in which we arrive damaged or we get damaged in our life-prospects during the course of our life's trajectory. Our lives are like rockets (or, if you like it better, like birds); some of us are getting shot down all the time.

Only Survivors Get To Be Old

Within this perspective or intellectual map of life's span, Old Age is just the plateau of life's wisdom and a time of very gradually ebbing energies. Old Age is that time in life in which the real survivors in life, having survived so much so well from the earlier decades, finally get their turn at what sometimes can be some very hard knocks.

Time-passing is not happening exclusively to us. It is happening also to the young. It is just that they will get to stay on a little longer than we.

But even so, Old Age is special for everyone who has the good luck and the privilege of surviving to enjoy it. Old Age induces in us a lingering nostalgia, for we know what we have liked about this life—and we can see it is gradually passing from us. But it is also passing from everyone else that is alive; time-passing is not happening exclusively to us. It is happening also to the young. It is just that they will get to stay on a little longer than we.

So I think that a more adequate intellectual map of our life span has to tell us that Old Age is really a very mixed bag with much that is good and some that is bad. In this respect Old Age is a lot like all the other decades and periods in our lifetime.

What seems vitally important is that we distinguish between Old Age (a period of time in our lives) and our exiting or our demise, our dying (the last moment of our lives). Exiting comes last, and for almost everyone dying is the pits.

But my observation of my mother and other Alzheimer's patients I know is that their illness seems to spare them our awareness of death. Blessedly they seem to forget death as well as much else in life. But that seems only fair. There have simply got to be some things on the benefit side of the cost and benefit ledger of Alzheimer's disease. Forgetting to have the awareness (and perhaps the dread) of dying seems like a biggie, a big benefit that goes with the rest of Alzheimer's disease.

12.

A Loss of Focus

Rethinking Alzheimer's Disease

How do I think about Alzheimer's disease? How do I think about my mother, who has Alzheimer's? This is an important and practical question because *how* I think affects *what I do*.

What if we were consciously to make the choice to emphasize not how the Alzheimer's patient is different? What if instead we were to choose to think in ways that highlight how he or she is still *similar* to you and me and to the person the Alzheimer's patient used to be?

Suppose I consciously choose to think about Alzheimer's in a different way, a way that would *not* separate off some of us as "diseased" or afflicted—which leaves the rest of us feeling well and secure, thinking and feeling that we are fundamentally different?

In other words, what if we were consciously to make the choice to emphasize not how the Alzheimer's patient is different? What if instead we were to choose to think in ways that highlight how he or she is still *similar* to you and me and to the person the Alzheimer's patient used to be?

If we made such a change in our minds, then we would focus our thoughts and our behavior upon a life-companion who is constantly changing (just as we ourselves are changing). We then would *expect* change in the Alzheimer's patient. We would try to understand those changes and to respond in helpful ways to them. And we would try to ease their effects upon the patient, upon ourselves, and upon the ongoing relationship we were still feeling ourselves companioned and partnered in.

What such a change of mind does is make Alzheimer's become a fact for my mother and me, a difficult fact. But it helps me recognize that there is not yet a death sentence for her or for our relationship.

I then have to work along at doing the best I can at coping with my mother's Alzheimer's disease, just as my mother does. This means I see both of us continuing our life-long struggles to find what benefits and pleasures are possible at each phase of our lives. And we continue to work to avoid or minimize our life's ever-changing disadvantages, pains, and costs.

In this view we are all in life's predicaments together, and always engaged in trying to find what good in our lives and relationships is still there, still to be enjoyed, remaining yet to be savored.

The Core Problem

The core problem, as I see it in my own experience with my mother, is the loss of focus that goes with Alzheimer's disease. What my mother and I are experiencing together is our life becoming more and more blurred. It is not that the wider world itself fades away. For my mother and for me, everything about our relationship is simply becoming increasingly less clear and hence harder to remember. It is less precisely perceived and then less and less understood, and hence in many respects less manageable.

We who are still unimpaired by Alzheimer's often focus upon what happens to someone's memory during the disease. We notice the patient no longer remembers which pocket (if any) has the house key (or car key). Something done a few minutes ago is often (but not always) not remembered. The person with Alzheimer's can get lost easily, and when they are not in their most familiar contexts they risk not remembering where they are or how to get home. The Alzheimer's patient not only can lose any place-sense but also any usual sense of time (what day of the week or month today is, what year this is, or how old I am). All this blurs, becomes imprecise, and then gradually goes totally out of focus.

For my mother and for me, everything about
our relationship is simply becoming
. . . less precisely perceived
and then less and less understood, and
hence in many respects less manageable.

But I have a problem with memory loss as the major way we describe Alzheimer's. So far as I know, I do not now have Alzheimer's disease. But I have experienced all of these things in some degree myself at one time or another. This is not my experience all the time. But it is frequent enough that I (or my wife or my children) notice. We can be driving for a time down the highway talking intensely, and suddenly I don't know how close I am to the exit we want. I have lost touch with my spatial location; it is not that I have forgotten it but that it has blurred in my mind while my emotional and intellectual attention was elsewhere.

Similarly, I forget where the keys (or my eyeglasses) are. Why?—because I wasn't looking (at myself) when I put them away or put them down. I am aware I have acted to protect myself from myself in these regards in at least two ways. At first, I systematized where I put the keys. In the house they are *always* in one place. And when I am out or going out, they are *always* stored in another place that goes with me. So I use habitual procedures to cover for me when my attention is routinely going to be focused upon other things.

My alternative strategy is to "up" my attention level. I found I was not really listening (attending to what was being said) when I was forgetting what my wife or one of our children had said to me about something. I now know (when I need to or want to) that I can grasp the spotlight of my emotional involvement and focus it more intensely and precisely. Otherwise, I may literally be focusing my attention elsewhere, as I think we all often do when we are driving a car over a familiar route or during a long trip on a superhighway. I am then often giving only apparent or superficial attention to what is outwardly "right in front of my eyes."

I know I am not alone in functioning out of focus.

At home, when my wife calls to me, I may be listening to someone else on the phone. If I am not on the phone I may be reading someone else's words (rather than hearing them). I have observed that under these circumstances I can hear the sound of my wife's words with my ears but I may not really be hearing her with my attention. A moment later I know she said *something,* but I really wasn't paying attention and often I cannot tell you (or myself) *what* she said.

Or I may be writing at my computer and listening intently to myself as I think and write. Then too my ears hear my wife's voice and I know (for example) that I have been called to dinner. But nowadays we have agreed that my wife does not expect she has really gotten my attention until, when she speaks, I utter a response, an answer, and make some commitment of attention to her and to our relationship.

I know I am not alone in functioning out of focus in this way. My wife is a feminist theologian, and she has observed that women report that what they often like most about love-making is not the final outcome but the journey to getting there. And central to that love-making journey is really having our beloved's full attention. The lover's and the beloved's thoughts and emotions and attention are stimulated, aroused, caught up in a high-resolution focus. Other concerns are pushed to the periphery as we center together upon the immediacy of this encounter.

We experience similarly intense focus outside the bedroom when we for a span of time are completely involved physically and mentally in playing some competitive sport. Or we are intensely engaged with a partner in a game of bridge or chess. If then a baby cries out or the phone rings, this is not only an intrusion into any of these occasions of high concern but it is disruptive. It is a minor "instantaneous transformation" that derails the entire emotional, intellectual, erotic process to a much inferior state. Yes, it is possible to start again, but it is "again." The moment is now gone. That special focus has been lost.

Dividing Our Attention, Orchestrating It, Relaxing It

So we all have experiences similar to Alzheimer's patients who are functioning with a loss of focus. But their loss is gradual and progressive, and without the option of "agains." Many of our ordinary day-to-day moments are far removed from our creative highs of concentration, attention and focus. In most ordinary moments we get along with a far more relaxed hold on life. We can and often do divide our attention among several activities or streams of conscious awareness and thought. We juggle these several mental states more or less all at once. We are like someone frequently switching TV channels in order to keep abreast of several programs simultaneously.

So we drive over a daily commuter route in our car, shifting lanes in familiar patterns. We are also perhaps aware of the car radio playing music or the news. Many of us are at the same time also lost in "planning" or thought, enjoying the intensity of our own inmost reflections.

Then suddenly something jars us into awareness of danger, and that experience gives us a glimpse within of still another layer of consciousness. What we have experienced is the arising within us of the occasional red flag of caution: "This road may be approaching the freezing point and suddenly become treacherous to stop on," or some similar warning to us.

When we are well, we enjoy our
having this capacity to cope with complexity
and to move as appropriate
among diffuse and multiple levels of focus.
But Alzheimer's disease
involves all this gradually coming unglued.

These diversified and even diffuse awarenesses of life are what many of us function with most of the time. Certainly a woman (or a man) getting dinner—with children in the background and listening to the radio or to TV news, preparing food, setting the table, and, at the same time, keeping track of the different times required for cooking several things on and in the stove, and also juggling all of the above to get everyone and everything to the table at the same time—is working with a lot.

But mostly we do not think about the complex and multilayered consciousness our lives sometimes require. We take all this quite for granted and we see it as simply how we live at some points, juggling several things at once and adjusting our priorities moment by moment.

When We Lose Our Concentration

When we are well, we enjoy our having this capacity to cope with complexity and to move as appropriate among diffuse and multiple levels of focus. Sometimes, when it is needed or desired, we shift to single-minded attention. Other times we are able to let go of attentiveness and simply enjoy an overall relaxation of all focus, what we know as the joy and restoration of sleeping or dozing.

But Alzheimer's disease involves all this gradually coming unglued. Try as we will, we cannot muster the appropriate focus, the needed attention. Lacking any longer the capacity to provide it for ourselves, we need to have the focus and attention to our life provided for us from outside. It needs to come from another person or from the planned structure of our environment, so that the normal functions and protections in our lives still work for us. My mother still gets hungry and needs to eat, but she is dependent on others to plan and prepare meals and now even to feed her enough to keep her going. She clearly still enjoys her food and its variety and it being appropriately hot (or cold) rather than tepid.

It is not that they are forgetting; I see many daily evidences that they remember, both yesterday and yesteryears. What seems lacking is the emotional energy to hold any of this in steady focus.

I notice her loss of focus especially with regard to sounds and what she hears. She and I can be talking and someone can speak in the next room or outside in the hall or, when we are in the common room, across the room. It is for her as though every voice, every sound, is equally intended for her attention and her response. Her hearing is still excellent, so in the midst of telling me something, if she hears someone ask a question, she will try to answer it. Often it is clear from the garbled state of her in and out communication that what she caught was not the substance of the question but the inflection and the urgency in the voice of the questioner.

It is as though everything now for her is in the foreground of her attention. Nothing is background or middleground. Everything is equally present, equally immediate in its demand upon her. In this overwhelming immediacy everything is important, everything is "now."

This seems a more comprehensive account of what I see happening to my mother and her Alzheimer friends and to their memories. It is not that they are forgetting; I see many daily evidences that they remember, both yesterday and yesteryears. What seems lacking is the emotional energy to hold any of this in steady focus. They are awash in a sea of immediacy in which everything just happens and nothing any longer can really be controlled or understood very well, focused well, or made to do what well-being and autonomy and responsibility taught all of us to take for granted in our former lives.

My mother's problem with immediacy thus is vastly different from ours, and so it is often difficult for us to sympathize with and even comprehend her problem.

Immediacy

So my mother with her Alzheimer's has a problem that not only confuses her but is confusing to us who are around her. We who think of ourselves as well are confused because actually attaining sufficient immediacy is a problem we all live with daily. Our minds and attentions are often on other things. Modern life encourages, even demands, that we juggle many layers of consciousness and complexity. A high-resolution focus on the immediate or now is rare for us.

My mother's problem with immediacy thus is vastly different from ours, and so it is often difficult for us to sympathize with and even comprehend her problem. She is awash in the present moment; whatever comes to her senses—whatever someone says to her, what she hears someone say to someone else, or what she overhears being said on the TV—*that* is the center of her moment. Or alternatively, the center of her moment may be whatever comes to her from within, from the depths of her own consciousness—a thought fragment, a memory, an idea, a comment, a feeling in response to whatever the present moment brings to her from outside or up from within.

The larger mental pictures we all
share with one another about the world
beyond our reach, seem to be
in the process of washing out of her mind.
They seem like old photographs that are fading.

All this seems to float still in an ongoing stream or flow of consciousness (just as the content of your moments and mine do). But in my mother's life it seems now to happen without much psychic "glue" holding it together.

When early in her Alzheimer's my mother was hospitalized for a week, she found that experience very confusing. What happened was that she no longer had any concept of "hospital," so "nurse" and "call button" were concepts far beyond her ken. So far as she knew she was still at home, except all the people were changed and the room was new and her life seemed transformed. She had a very disoriented week in the hospital, during which we tried to spend a great deal of time reassuring her just by our presence with her. When she came home to her familiar setting, she clicked back into old surroundings and known people—and she seemed again her only slightly confused early-Alzheimer's self. At that point she had just sufficient psychic "glue" to cope with the familiar— but not with the unfamiliar.

In my mother's Alzheimer's disease, the larger mental pictures we all share with one another about the world beyond our reach, seem to be in the process of washing out of her mind. They seem like old photographs that are fading. Hence her capacity to make sense of her life and of such experiences as the hospital was clearly diminishing, in what was for her an alarming way.

The "now" where my mother lives is really where all our living is taking place.

Yet the Alzheimer's patients I see have a tranquility and peacefulness amid it all that their actual circumstances scarcely justify. I know there are good pharmaceuticals available to soften their anxieties, though I have no way of knowing who is medicated with what. As we get acquainted, what strikes me most is their gentleness, their grace, their continuing efforts to work at the elements they can in the daily game of life. Some walk and walk and walk. Some work away at using their wheelchairs to keep their mobility. My mother talks, and it is from her talking (whether I or anyone else is talking back) that I realize how much alive my mother still is in her succession of moments as she strings them loosely together, one tumbling after another. All is present and immediate. Little is yesterday, still less is tomorrow. Like the other Alzheimer's patients around her, she is busy making her peace with the present moment. And, for this time in her life, that is sufficient.

Look at our "well" lives for a moment. Despite all our "well" thoughts (and worries) about tomorrow and about our yesterdays, do *we* really do it much differently? The "now" where my mother lives is really where all our living is taking place. The rest is our participation in a vast shared cultural construction of reality. It is a vast shared work of mind and imagination, our explanation of it all to one another and to ourselves. What she has lost is those explanations and the emotional energy or "glue" that holds them together. What keeps her going now is the living itself.

13.

Talking to Garble

Settling Down to Boredom

It has been four or five months since I have written about my mother. It has been a difficult time for her, for me, for us. We have settled down into familiarity, into tedium, into endless repetitions that seem to be part of an infinite series each like the other, yet slightly different, sometimes slightly better, sometimes slightly worse.

Always her face lights up when I appear in the common room. I am grateful that she recognizes me, though the other night I got an insight into how fragile that recognition is. It was one of her better evenings of late for conversation, and as we struggled along seeking to understand one another in between the spoonfuls of her supper that I was helping her with, my mother asked me, "How is your mother?"

I thought I had learned to take in stride whatever comes, but this instant in time stopped me in my tracks. First I covered for her, playing back to her a conversation of pleasant concern: "She's doing very well," I said. But I could not contain those feelings and that charade; I burst into a broad grin at my mother and said to her, "*You're* my mother."

"Oh yes," she smiled, with what I recognized (I thought) as a tinge of cunning or knowing, and she continued chewing.

As Winter Settles In Upon Us

This incident implies more conversation than we have been having in recent months. It goes back to that time of season in November when in New England we settle into darkness so early in the evening.

It has been a difficult time for her, for me, for us. We have settled down into familiarity, into tedium, into endless repetitions that seem to be part of an infinite series.

I would arrive by walking from our house across the playing fields through total darkness, accompanied only by stars if the sky was clear, stars and the distant sounds of commuter traffic rushing homebound on the highway. The energy of life seems to me at a low ebb then anyhow, and we draw into the warmth of our homes and relationships, pull the curtains and prepare our dinners with the sense that the outer world is less hospitable. We need the warmth and personal energy of our homes and our bundled-up winter clothing to help us through these times.

Perhaps I was bringing these sentiments with me to my mother as I came in from my brisk walk through the dark. But whatever the source of my perception of her, she seemed to me to be gradually fading away, a super–slow-motion version of what happens to the television image when the power is turned off in a dark room. The image collapses and for a minute or so a ghost-image lingers on the tube and then is finally gone.

One evening as we were at supper I asked Cissy or Laurie as staff where Clara Jacobs was. As I looked around the common room I didn't see her. "She died last night in her sleep," I was told.

It was happening, I realized anew. It was as though Clara had somehow gotten up in the night and, instead of simply getting out of her bed and bedding, one way or another she got out of her body. And she walked out into the ebbing energy of the coming winter and its long night. A deep shudder of recognition went through me, chilling my spine. I was so glad I was having these last hours, days, minutes, with my mother, for I knew as dimly she must too, that her time to slip out was coming.

The Illness

Several weeks later I found a message on my telephone-answering device. "Mr. Gray, your mother has an elevated temperature this morning. We have called the doctor. Will you please phone us right away." My heart sank. Is this it? I wondered.

They had reached my mother's physician. They were beginning antibiotics immediately, and everything seemed under control for the moment. I went immediately and saw my mother briefly. She was lying in her bed, the sides up. I don't remember whether the television was going quietly in the background to keep her company. She no longer felt hot with fever to my touch but the brightness was out of her eyes and she seemed listless and without any desire to communicate or be companioned. I came back at dusk and she was in a deep sleep. I stood by her bed for perhaps a minute, listening to my mother's breathing and to the background noises of the nursing home and staff and to my mother's "neighbors" as they went on about the now familiar routines of the supper-hour. Her steady breathing and deep sleep seemed healing, and I left quietly.

The next evening I was astonished to find my mother sitting up in her special reclining chair on wheels in the common room. She ate her supper that night with veritable gusto. I realized that she had eaten little for twenty-four hours or more. But she seemed to spring back from that long deep sleep of the evening before, and I was very grateful for her vigor and the prompt care from the staff of the nursing home.

The Aftermath

But all was not over.

I gradually became aware that the day-to-day variations in my mother's capacities to relate to me while I was helping her with her dinner had dropped half a note, shifted for the worse so that, while her trend of well-being did not seem to be downward, nonetheless it was not as good as it had been during the summer and fall.

When I compared this September with a year ago
I knew she was worse, substantially worse.

"She's getting worse," I thought, and I felt another wave of dread moving over me, again at super-slow pace. Everything seemed to happen so slowly, so gradually, even my awareness of her changes amid the day-to-day ups and downs. I had known with my mind that her condition could only degrade, but for so long she had seemed to hang on with such spirit and even determination. Yes, when I compared this September with a year ago I knew she was worse, substantially worse. When I compared her condition today with that of the other women patients who had lunch with us at a special table on the occasion of my mother's first meal at the nursing home, I had still another standard for comparison.

Clara Jacobs was already gone. But Wilma and Kate, as well as my mother, are still here. Wilma is in a wheelchair always. Kate is even better off, for she can get up and get about with her walker when she feels like it. It is clear that my mother's condition has deteriorated in the year at a faster rate than Wilma's and Kate's. With Clara already gone, my mother seems to be next. I wonder, does she calculate such things too?

I look around the common room now and I realize that, over time, I have come to know everyone here and they me. A part of it is my being here every evening when I am not away traveling. But it is also that some have worsened, gotten feebler, moved from a wheelchair to reclining-chair-with-wheels (such as my mother now lives in) or finally moved to their bed, or to the more intensive nursing care of the other unit. Or they have died. And a new class, they are almost the freshmen here, has entered. They walk about more, talk better, get homesick, their families come to visit, a few have regular visits each evening at supper time. There is a gradual changeover in the makeup of our community of patients, staff, and attending family-members.

My mother's sudden illness heightened my perceptions of all these changes. After all, it was a year now that she had lived here, a year of dinner hours that I had spent with her. It has been a lot of precious last-times.

Widening My Participation in My Mother's World

By early February of her second year in the nursing home I had become accustomed to my mother not being able to communicate with me very much over her supper. I found this more boring for me, as perhaps it was also for her. Gradually I took more part in the general common room discussion during dinner. This was generated by the staff and the more mobile or more vocal patients. The phonograph would be playing dinner music in the background, and the staff would react verbally to one or another of the patients. It was akin to banter but it was more kindly and supportive. It was a job for the staff but they also knew and cared for these old (and not so old) people. They knew them well and could draw them out emotionally as well as verbally.

The staff also talked with one another at this time. About the late-movie one of them had watched the night before. Or about plans and frustrations connected with a winter holiday coming up soon in the sunny Caribbean. Or about me, as they came to include me in their circle and got to satisfy their curiosity about who I was and what I did. In turn they told me gradually about the former accomplishments of some of my mother's neighbors. This one was a painter and had written a book with her husband, a physician. She had been actively painting as recently as three years ago, I was told. Another was a physician, another a banker. I realized that only a few years separated them from us, a decade or more if we are lucky. This is one way to be old, not the only way, but certainly a common one.

I came back from a trip of a week's duration in early February and was astounded. My mother's capacity for communication had sprung back. She was more alive, vital, concerned, talkative. On the phone I told her cousin Karl that I thought I had made a mistake about her condition. What I realized now was that my mother had been exhausted, dragged down by her bout of illness in mid-December and it had taken her six weeks to two months to regain her energies.

Talking to Garble

My mother had not been uncommunicative during her recovery. It was just, I could now see, that she had not had the energy to spare for projecting a conversation. She could not push at life and make very many demands that it conform to what she wanted. She had gone limp and seemed to me very much more withdrawn and passive.

She still could not take great initiatives. Whereas earlier I had learned to "listen to garble," now I was learning to "talk to garble." This was a more difficult skill, and it built upon the previous one. Now, I realized, I was having to carry even more of the conversation. But I had to carry it in a different way, for increasingly I had not the slightest idea what my mother was trying to tell me. What was I to do?

I realized that I could respond to my mother's implied emotion. One evening, for example, she garbled something to me and the only word I could distinguish was the unusual word *joke*. It was also clear from the inflection of the ending of her sentence that my mother had asked me a question. In my imagination I created a possible sentence: Would I like her to tell me a joke?

I laughed and said, "Of course I would like to hear a joke."

My mother garbled and garbled and garbled. It was a joke with a context which she had to create, and then there must have been a punch line, for she ended her account quite decisively and with a large smile on her face. And I laughed; we laughed together. It was a precious moment. My mother was never known for her sense of humor; I have no memories of her ever previously having told a joke in my hearing. But she had told me a joke now, and it was a good moment for us both. I shall never be able to retell that joke, nor do I understand the content of it at all. But it was clear to us both what had happened. My mother had wanted to tell me a joke, I had been able to imagine what she wanted from such meager clues, and we had enjoyed a moment of joke-telling (if not an actual joke) together.

Now, I realized, I was having to carry even more of the conversation, and in a different way, for increasingly I had not the slightest idea what my mother was trying to tell me.

What had also happened was that I had "talked" to her garble in such a way as to allow, or even encourage, my mother to make the effort to communicate with me. It is experiences such as this which make me think there is more mental functioning still going on inside of her than she is now able to express. It seems to me akin to problems we all have occasionally with our telephones when we are calling someone and they can hear us but we cannot hear them. Or vice versa. What we do when the problem is technological is to redial the call. There is no such technological option with my mother. The communication seems also to be garbled in-bound as well as out-bound. But amid the garble there are individual word-fragments and sometimes entire out-of-context sentences which are intelligible. It is to these that I try to speak.

It is experiences such as this which make me think there is more mental functioning still going on inside of her than she is now able to express.

Talk That Is Enabling

When my mother asked me, "How is your mother?" I had two alternatives. I realize now that, being her son, I was emotionally involved in that particular confusion and I responded from my own need to clarify who we were for one another. It is also possible that what she really meant to ask me was about my wife. In reaching to name that important woman in my life, perhaps the closest she could come was "mother." My mother when she was starting her Alzheimer's disease was aware Liz was having some health problems; while she sees me almost daily, perhaps she has wondered why she has not been seeing Liz. Sometimes I do tell her about Liz and update her on how she is doing. But also of course my mother forgets.

My point is that sometimes when my mother tries to communicate, I respond from *my* need for emotional satisfaction rather than by playing back to *her* need to communicate. My most helpful talking with my mother takes place when I am able to concentrate upon enabling her communication.

Doing this involves me in making imaginative reconstructions from sometimes very meager clues about my mother's intentions. Sometimes it is just one word in a sentence, such as the name of her cousin ("Karl") or her sister ("Ruth") or the simple word "Mother." Often all I have to go on is this one word, plus listening to the inflection (Is this a question, or is this a declarative statement?). And often I can hear her emotion (Is this being said in a tentative and questioning mode, or is something being passionately felt and communicated?).

Sometimes when my mother tries to communicate, I respond from my need for emotional satisfaction rather than by playing back to her need to communicate. My most helpful talking with my mother takes place when I am able to concentrate upon enabling her communication.

Sometimes talking to garble involves responding only to the inflection (when that is all that is clear). For example, my mother is asking me a question (from the inflection) but not a single word is anything but garble. In these circumstances I may say, "Do you think I should know?" or perhaps another time I will say, "I don't know either. I wonder if anyone knows." The first response elicits further information from my mother; the latter response has the emotional impact of my standing alongside her in her not-knowing. Both responses tend to encourage her to say more to me, to keep trying, and to feel that in me she has a sympathetic ally.

I have listened with amazement as the staff around my mother do this with other patients. It is clear (to me) that Cissy and Laurie are listening to extremely scant clues and making enormous imaginative efforts in their attempts to reconstruct a possible meaning which might make sense for this patient and this particular communication. I note also with awe the ease with which they reach out to caress a face, to make gentle physical contact, as they try to talk to garble, to reassure a patient that attentive caring has been elicited, and to express the enjoyment that frequently is there in such moments.

Imagining That Helps

Talking to garble is an increased act of imagination beyond listening to garble. It involves a much increased act of imagination beyond what we are all accustomed to in trying to understand one another in usual conversation. But talking to garble really is possible. Sometimes it works better than other times. It may work better this time because we are given more cues to work with. And sometimes our imagining seems more inspired than at other times. But it is a skill; we can work at learning it and then at improving it. And the progressive deterioration which characterizes Alzheimer's disease continues apace, and most of the time our skills barely stay abreast of it.

Talking to garble is an increased act of imagination beyond listening to garble.
It involves a much increased act of imagination beyond what we are all accustomed to in trying to understand one another in usual conversation.

But talking to garble is imaginative listening-and-caring that really helps. It helps the person with Alzheimer's even if only in their sense that we are paying careful attention and continuing to try to take their communications seriously. My own experience is that this skill also helps me when I am talking with all those who do not have Alzheimer's. As I learn to "listen to" and "talk to" the garble of Alzheimer's, I am amazed at how I now detect garble in other communications. We can make better responses to many of the everyday communications if we use our newly developed skills at "imagining that helps" and let these skills guide both our understanding and our responses.

We have all known for a long time that much we hear is not very clear, has lots of hidden messages, and otherwise baffles us. Alzheimer's garble is just more of the same. But now it is coming from someone we love, and it is worth trying seriously in this instance to listen and to respond.

14.

Night Work

A Bittersweet Time

I have been aware of an unusual feeling of being depressed. I am lethargic, not doing things that need doing or doing them not on schedule. For several nights I woke up aware of a vague dis-ease or diffuse anxiety. It is now early summer and it has been a long time since I have wanted to write about my mother and her Alzheimer's. Instead I have simply spent time with her each day,

---

A veritable landslide has occurred which has taken away so much of her capability.

---

helping her eat her evening meal, supporting her efforts to communicate by emotionally sensing her intentions and attempting empathetically to mirror back to her appropriate if often vague responses. Just looking around the common room where she spends most of her days, I can see that, as she reclines comfortably in her special geriatric chair-on-wheels, she has moved from what my wife recently characterized as "freshman" status (newcomer) to being right up there with the "seniors," those most advanced in disability. This happens slowly, so slowly you can't see it happening. But when I remember early winter nineteen months ago when she arrived here, and also where she was, by my own accounts, a year ago, I am sobered. It has been rapid; a veritable landslide has occurred which has taken away so much of her capability.

My mother is still there to me; her face lights up when I appear or when I touch her cheek. She is emotionally as responsive as ever. But I feel as though the communication channels, both inbound and as she communicates outward, become less and less accessible to us both. It is a bittersweet time, and I think we both know it.

I wonder, and I know Liz at her worst moments does too, whether Liz might die of a recurrence of her cancer before Mom dies of her Alzheimer's.

The Balancing Act

I find I am learning a balancing act. Or I have been doing one during these months of springtime and now early summer. My wife Liz is more recuperated from her own three and a half years of painful physical therapy, and just in time. Her professional life is resurrecting itself with her help. She is getting speaking engagements again, so that this spring has been busy and next fall will be hectic, with Liz traveling in October most weeks twice a week, sometimes two distant round-trip flights in one week. I have been traveling with her this spring when the destinations are close enough for us to choose to drive, so that she could have access to my aid and also my physical therapy skills to deal with pain, should it occur, without having to let it crescendo from neglect until she could get home to me.

So there have been choices to be with Liz which mean my not being with Mom. Sometimes this is only for two days or three, but on occasion it has meant not being with my mother for five or six evening meals—a long time in her life. I have wondered if I overestimate my importance to her days. Or to her nutrition, for I know I can take longer to feed her and get her to eat more than most of the regular staff can. I know she keeps eating for me because she knows that when she stops, I will go. She's still no fool; she is disabled but not foolish! I know also how much her speech improves when I am there for half an hour; at the start she is quite unfocused, and by the end there is genuine dialogue, if not complete communication. I am bringing her more than nutrition; I provide the daily occasion to come back to emotional focus by the attention I can give and the occasion for motivation I can provide. When I come back after being away for a number of days, I can see the difference, I think, and I feel as though I am having to reach further down into some well to help her struggle back out.

But I am balancing her needs against Liz'. I wonder, and I know Liz at her worst moments does too, whether Liz might die of a recurrence of her cancer before Mom dies of her Alzheimer's. I am aware of juggling—of balancing; and as Liz' capacity to bloom professionally opens up again with these speaking engagements, I am choosing to support Liz over Mom. But I think a lot about Mom, and when Liz can be home resting at that for-us pre-dinner hour while I help Mom, I am pleased to be able to choose to support both of them.

What has become so vivid for us is our memory of the years while our children were still at home for Christmas, home from school, home from college. We had not been foresighted enough to realize that soon Lisa would be in San Diego (and now in Santa Barbara) a continent away, and Hunter in Washington, D.C. and soon in Utah—and our Christmases together with them here would be gone forever. We were all aware that Mom was growing older, and we had delighted after Dad's death to transport our Christmases to her Florida home. Then, after she moved back to Rhode Island, it seemed natural to be with her there on Christmas Day. What we did was rush through our time together with our children, putting our Christmases under great time-stress. We did this because we expected our Christmases with Mom to be few and therefore special. What we had not anticipated was that our Christmases with our children were also few and running out, and also special.

Had we realized then what we know now, we simply would have shuffled the times around differently. We would have planned for two separate celebrations of Christmas, and allowed ample time and separation for each of them. But we failed to notice that we were balancing, juggling, and so we dropped out of our lives special Christmas experiences and occasions with our children which we knew even then were important to us all. The irony is that Mom herself would have agreed with this assessment.

To be living with all this mortality-stuff and incorporating it into everyday decisions about what to do next, does take its daily toll. I experienced this toll in my dreams as I slept.

The Dream

What we know now is that we have to be paying attention constantly to the needs and opportunities of each of the generations, Mom, ourselves as the middle generation, and our children. And we must know that we cannot assume immortality and no surprises for any of us. But it does take its daily toll to be living with all this mortality-stuff and incorporating it into everyday decisions about what to do next. I experienced this toll in my dreams as I slept.

When I was coming awake on a recent morning I was aware of awakening also from a dream. It was an unusual dream because my mother was in it. My remembrance of the dream is that it is already in process. There are earlier dream events now forgotten, and my memory of the dream begins with me standing in a line waiting to fill a dinner plate at a buffet. No one is carving the leg of roast beef as I would expect at a usual buffet, and each of us is having to do it ourselves. I am getting through the line very slowly, and I am aware I am filling the plate not for myself but for my mother. As we wait in line I am complaining to my neighbor about this system.

Suddenly I am driving my car and I am stopped in heavy traffic. I decide I can help my mother with her day-trip into New York City by exiting to the railroad station and picking up a train schedule and her ticket. In retelling the dream later to Liz, I recalled that recently one of the volunteers at the nursing home told me of going with three other staff members and five patients on a several-hour cruise of Boston Harbor to enjoy the summer breezes and the change and the ocean views. But in my dream the day-trip for my mother was to be to New York City.

The traffic was slow, stop-and-go. Finally I got out and, like pulling a child's sled by its rope, I was able to pull my car by a rope through an opening in the traffic into the parking lot of a suburban railroad station. (We walk nightly by a similar rail station for commuters going into Boston.)

But I realized I was apprehensive. Would my mother really feel secure getting off a train in Grand Central Station in New York, being in the City for a few hours, and then getting herself back to the station and onto a return train? I quietly reversed my decision to buy her ticket and otherwise help her with arrangements for her outing.

Then I woke up. The dream would have gone on, but it did not because I returned to my waking world.

Listening to the Language of Dreams

One of the things Liz and I do, while getting our day started by bathing, dressing, and having breakfast together, is to talk about our dreams whenever we awaken with them. What I found most striking was that after this dream I awoke feeling better. I told Liz about my dream and what I took to be its effect upon my inner climate of feelings. I interspersed the associations and connections from my awake-world to that dream's world pretty much as I have recounted them here.

"What," Liz asked me, "do you think the whole dream was about?" I saw its parts but I had not been able to see it as a whole, so I told her I was not sure.

"I think," she said, "you have been dreaming not about your mother's trip into a New York City which she could not handle, but into her dying. You have been helping her slog through the slow succession of days by feeding her—the delays in the buffet line and then in the traffic jam. You knew she was going to take a trip you were apprehensive about. Your first reaction was to help her with it by picking up her ticket. But then you decided the trip wouldn't be good for her so you changed your mind.

"And when you got close to your mother's dying, you woke up, exited the situation. The dreaming broke off when it got too close to the pain it was trying to handle."

Today I awoke from still another long dream with similar themes. But the dream-deck had been shuffled, so to speak, and came out in still another way. I was at a conference center in the mountains and a part of my necessary gear was some distance away at another facility. Liz and I would have to drive there quickly to fetch it and return. Someone pointed out to me the place I needed to go, far up and atop a distant high hill or mountain.

We were driving quickly there when suddenly I realized we were coming over the crest and were about to go suddenly down over the mountainside into a very deep chasm. I stopped. We then drove off in the car in another direction, and soon we were having a similar experience. We came quickly up to a crest in the road and saw the roadway suddenly end and go off a precipice into another steep mountain ravine.

Then we were back at the original conference site. I had retrieved what I needed and we were in a worship service. Suddenly I as a minister was standing and leading people in prayer, holding them close in my arms. What I felt coming from my lips and heart were deeply meaningful words and imagery of authentic supplications to God about our own mortality, and concerns about death being in our midst and about dying. It felt so very good to me to find these words and these images in which to be able to express what was so very painful for us all. The words of my prayer felt as though they were a great release of pain and feeling for everyone.

And again I awoke to my daytime life.

In all probability there will be more such dreams fashioned by my sleeping self to catch the emotional overflow of my waking life. I feel as though the beginnings of an emotional logjam in my inner self has begun to break up.

Today I am refreshed, no longer lethargic, and my moments are no longer surrounded by a penumbra of depression. Tonight I will again be with my mother for dinner, and for many more tonights and dinners, I hope. I know that in all probability there will be more such dreams fashioned by my sleeping self to catch the emotional overflow of my waking life. I feel as though the beginnings of an emotional logjam in my inner self has begun to break up. My sleeping self is finally becoming able to help my waking self process some of the deeply-held emotions I have been unable to feel and to face in my waking life.

I do not always like my dream life. There was terror in suddenly coming to the end of the roadway and stopping just short of the edge of a ravine. But those apparently are the feelings my awake self has been unable to face and cope with, and my sleeping self which I count on each night to knit up the ravelled sleeve of body energy is also able to knit up the ravelled sleeve of these cares. I am very grateful for that wonderful versatility of my sleeping self. I will need it often in the weeks or months ahead.

Part 3.

Home at Last

15.

Toward the Finish Line

Running the Race

My mother died nine months later on the 18th of March. She would have been eighty-four in June. It is now nearly two months later. The tulips are in bloom, the flowering cherry trees and crabapples are in full display, and I see all around me the tokens of another season and another generation of life coming to be. Still, my days and dreams at night are tinged with sadness, a soft sorrow that recedes when I am caught up in other activities or relationships but which is always there, not going away.

I feel as though my mother in her Alzheimer's
was making her way slowly
down a very long corridor with no doors;
the first exit-door she came to, she took.

I have told innumerable people in person, by note, on the phone, that I feel as though my mother in her Alzheimer's was making her way slowly down a very long corridor with no doors; the first exit-door she came to, she took. Others of her neighbors had died, some suddenly, some gradually. In January Kate stopped eating. Her Alzheimer's disease had been proceeding at a slower pace than my mother's. Although Kate and my mother were in similar condition when my mother first came, gradually my mother had outpaced Kate in the race toward some unseen finish line. Then quite suddenly for a few weeks Kate found the determination to not eat and to die. My mother continued on, the round of her days uninterrupted and perhaps her morale sustained by our dinnertimes together and the loving concern of Cissy and Laurie and the other staff.

Then suddenly and unexpectedly in late February my mother faltered. She had had colds before. She had even run a temperature and stayed in bed for a day. But always before she bounced back in a few days and slowly resumed the race she was on. It must have seemed to her like a marathon, something that was endless and that she was running one way or another her whole life long. Her Alzheimer's, I am sure, felt to her like what long distance runners describe as "hitting the wall," the point at which you must go on but you no longer have the resources in you to do it, but you do.

My mother began to cough. In between mouthfuls of food she went into a spasm of chest-wrenching as she reached for her next breath. Then she would somehow get control of her breathing, shift her lungs or her chest so as to avoid the spot that provoked the difficulty, and go on. Some nights she would eat only a mouthful or two (I wondered if it was to please me) before she would decide that if the choice was between eating (and pleasing me) or the convulsion of coughing, she would not eat. We shifted to a nutritionally fortified milk shake which she could drink, and she did.

I came in one evening to find my mother not in the common room with the others but in her own room. She was on oxygen to help her breathing; her lungs had begun to fill up. The nurse could take her off the oxygen, I would feed her some and talk with her. In about half an hour her lungs would begin to fill, the coughing would return, and Cissy would use a nasal tube to empty her lungs. The portable suction machine was now always by her bedside. It was an exhausting experience for my mother, being suctioned. But then she could go back on the oxygen and feel better. She could rest now, breathing more shallowly but getting enough air without provoking her coughs.

Respite

I was amazed the next evening to find my mother back in the common room. She was restored, back onto the trajectory of a week or month ago. She had thrown off her coughing, her lungs had cleared themselves, and she was back up and running with the others in the pack. She had recovered from a touch of pneumonia, I thought.

"No," I said, "that's not appropriate. Hospitals are for life-extension, and that is not what is called for here."

A few days or a week later her lungs began to fill again. We repeated the cycle but over a longer period of time. There was a replacement nurse on duty one Sunday night, one from the nursing-temporaries agency. She was young. I asked her when she had a minute to come help my mother with some suctioning. She came in a few minutes. As she was preparing the nasal tube she said to me, "This is getting more and more frequent; we may need to have her go to the hospital for a workup and find out what's going on."

I amazed myself with my response.

"No," I said, "that's not appropriate. Hospitals are for life-extension, and that is not what is called for here."

I forget what her response was. She suctioned my mother, put her on oxygen again, and my mother and I settled into the relief of her being able to breathe easily once again without her struggling over her coughing. In a few minutes the week-end nursing supervisor appeared at my mother's door and beckoned to me. I had known her in a casual way over many months; we knew each other's names and she knew I was a regular feature of dinner-hour in the common room.

Outside in the hall we talked, out of earshot of my mother. Her opening words were reassuring: "I understand completely your concern." She told me she had gone through this a few months ago with one of her relatives. The nurse I had been talking to, I should understand, was an agency nurse and accustomed to working in hospitals where saving lives was the whole point, not helping people as they ease out of this life.

I told her of my concern that my mother be kept as comfortable as could be; that several years earlier she had been in the hospital and found it very disorienting; and so far as my brother and I were concerned (he was in Texas but we had discussed this by phone) we felt our mother would want the first possible way out of her Alzheimer's disease. I went on to recall another patient who, some months earlier, had been rushed to the hospital several times at the family's insistence and then had died one night in her sleep from her heart problem. I had learned then from talking with the LPNs about the possibility of a DNR order—"Do Not Resuscitate." I recalled also parishioners I had known who, dying of cancer, had been brought back from heart attacks. I, we, did not want that for my mother.

"We can do a DNR," she said. "It requires a written order from her doctor, but I can start that process with a phone call right now. He will phone you this evening at home probably, and then he will come in and write up the order. I'll make certain," she said, "that everyone is clear about the change for your mother."

I went back and sat with my mother. I held her hand and we sat quietly. She was enjoying my company and the respite from coughing that the oxygen was giving her. She was a woman who always seemed to me to live mostly in the moment, responding to it, adapting and making the best of it, whatever "it" was. I wondered if she knew—if in such circumstances any of us knows or can imagine—the increasingly slippery slope she was now venturing on. I who was well could scarcely discern its possible outlines.

I wondered if she knew—
if in such circumstances any of us
knows or can imagine—
the increasingly slippery slope she
was now venturing on.

Like Jigsaw Puzzle Pieces

I walked home across the still-frozen playing fields that night deep in thought and feeling. I had identified as drawing nearer, for my mother and for me, a parting we all know is a certainty, but which we leave conveniently shrouded in uncertainty, not allowing our imaginations to play upon it or bring it to the fullest vision we are capable of. Our time of parting, and her departing this life, was something I had never allowed myself to dwell upon, to anticipate. I knew it was a generic reality, something that came eventually in one way or another to all relationships. But I had taken steps this evening to bring it about for my mother and to not prolong it for her when it came. It had come upon me so suddenly in the statement of that nurse and my response, and then in my conversation with the nursing supervisor. I was still catching up with what was taking place.

I talked with my brother by phone, telling him of our mother's condition, the conversation with the nurses, and making sure he was still in agreement about the DNR order. I was no sooner off the phone with him than the doctor phoned. I retold everything to him, ending with my just completed talk with my brother. And it was agreed: he would write the DNR order. He would add to it that she might be given morphine to calm her if she became agitated. I could feel several more elements slipping into place in my mental picture of what was coming for my mother. I thanked the doctor and we each hung up.

These times were like vitamin pills in the bottle: they were an indeterminate but finite (and small) number. Day by day we were using them up.

I did not sleep well. I do not remember my dreams of those nights, but I do remember talking with my wife, whose five surgeries for breast cancer had paralleled my mother's time with Alzheimer's disease. I told Liz I was realizing now what I had not allowed myself to imagine about her breast cancer. Throughout her surgeries and her long process of physical therapy I simply refused to think about Liz' dying. Liz had thought about it, dreamt about it, been sleepless about it. She told me many times how it was the last thing she thought about going to sleep—and sometimes the terror of it catapulted her right back to wakefulness, making actually getting down into sleep a precarious psychological maneuver. I knew also that in these years her first thought upon waking was of her own dying. Liz was living within this existential anxiety about her own mortality and I was not. I was solicitous, thoughtful, helpful. I stayed awake with her many nights (but not enough). But I did not think about death—her death, my death, or, until now, my mother's death.

Those defenses were now breaking down under the pressure of impending reality. My times with my mother over the supper hour were more filled with emotion and meaning than ever before. I knew in my heart that these times were like vitamin pills in the bottle: they were an indeterminate but finite (and small) number.

Day by day we were using them up. Would it be this week, several weeks, several months? I did not know, except I knew her end was coming. Now I knew it, could feel it, and it pressed upon me. These were precious times together; all times are precious times but I was brightly aware now of how precious, and few, these were to be.

Our Various Preparations

I talk with my mother about almost everything. But I did not talk with her about the DNR. She was present when the agency nurse and I had our back-and-forth about my mother going to the hospital and my saying, No, hospitals were for life-extensions and that wasn't appropriate. My memory is not clear on this point, but I think I must have been aware that my mother could have understood that exchange. I think it likely that in the time after the agency nurse left and before the nursing supervisor beckoned me into the hallway, I may very well have talked with my mother about my sense that it was inappropriate for her to go to the hospital; that I was sure she did not want that; and that hospitals were for life-extension, and that clearly was not what she wanted now.

My mother would not have been able to say anything to this; she was months past that. But her eyes and, yes, her mind as expressed in those eyes were still bright and clear and alert. Had she been upset by that exchange or by my comments, she could have let me know. I came back later that night just as the evening shift was being relieved by the night shift, what in industry they call the graveyard shift. The doctor had been in, the DNR order was written in my mother's medical orders, and my mother was sleeping peacefully without oxygen and without coughing. It would not be tonight, I thought, but it will be soon.

The days went by. My mother's body rallied and was able to absorb the fluid from her lungs. One of the nurses told me they had her on diuretics to help her pass more fluids. And she was getting a potassium supplement to make up for what was being leached from her body. My mother was clearly needing to struggle to keep her breathing and her eating from causing her to go into a spasm of coughing. But, as she had done for a lifetime, she found ways to adapt in her breathing and her eating, and she coughed very little even though, it seemed, the possibility was always there and she was guarding herself against it. We enjoyed being together much as we had before, I providing much of the conversation and my mother responding with her eyes, her expression, her touch to my hand in hers. It was a little eternity in the midst of time, a time as though there were no time passing. She was on the oxygen, then off, suctioned sometimes every half-hour, sometimes only a few times a day. Then she was on oxygen all the time.

These were without doubt some of our last hours,
even minutes, together. Anything I wanted
to tell my mother before we were parted
I had better start saying right now.

Her body was no longer keeping pace with the fluids that were filling her lungs. Her breathing was becoming increasingly shallow but by now she knew how to avoid the racking fits of coughing. Her eyes were no longer on me when I arrived, they no longer sparkled in welcome. Instead she lay in her bed, partly elevated at the head, her eyes staring fixedly at the ceiling. Small wonder the ancients thought the gaze of the dying was fixed upon a heaven above. I think instead my mother now found it too emotionally painful to become reengaged with me and with all in her life that she cared about and somehow intuited she was losing her grip upon. But whether she paid attention to me or not, I held her hand and kept her company. From time to time I spoke. Then it came to me that these were without doubt some of our last hours, even minutes, together. Anything I wanted to tell my mother before we were parted I had better start saying right now.

Last Words

I began by telling my mother what I thought was happening. I said I didn't know whether she understood what was going on in her body, but her lungs were filling up faster than her body could remove the fluids. She had pneumonia and I didn't think it was going to be too long now before her turn at life was going to end. I told her I wasn't sure whether it would be tonight or this week or several weeks. But it was not going to be long. I said much the same things two nights in a row, each time telling her at the end, as I was leaving, that I did not know whether she would be here in the morning but I would be back.

I told her that she had had a wonderful life and that I was so glad she had been my mother. She was a wonderful mother and I really appreciated all the love and support she had been to my brother and to me throughout our lifetimes. I reminded her of when her mother had died in her arms. She had had to carry on. And now it was coming to her turn to go. She had her two sons who would carry on, and she had four wonderful grandchildren following in the generation after us. It was like a relay race and you passed the baton on to those who come after.

I told her the winter frost outside was melting and it was going to be spring again soon. The cycle of the seasons will go on. You have enjoyed the coming of springtime and summer and winter for a lot of years; you've had your turn at life and it is nearly over for you now, I said. I told her then what people know about what happens when we die: when you go you are going to go to a bright warm wonderful light. And there you are going to be met and welcomed by someone you've been very close to who has already gone on ahead of you. I wonder, I said, if it will be Muthie (I used her favorite nickname for her mother). Or would it be Ruth (her nearly-twin sister she had been so very close to until she died of cancer nearly thirty years ago)?

I don't know how much of what I was saying she was actually getting. Was she listening as she gazed with such fixity at the ceiling of her room? Or was my voice like a radio-voice that one tries to repress when one is desperately trying to put oneself to sleep? I was convinced she could understand me now as much as she did for months when we had dinnertimes together as I fed her, talking all the time while she chewed and responded with her eyes and facial expressions.

Then the words and music of a Negro spiritual came into my mind and I started singing softly to her as I stroked her forehead and my warm tears welled up in my eyes and streamed from my cheeks onto hers. It was a tender moment together as I sang "Swing low, Sweet chariot, Coming for to carry me home; Swing low, Sweet chariot, Coming for to carry me home." I remembered some of the stanzas and those I forgot I just hummed until I got back to words I could sing. My mother was breathing rapidly and extremely shallowly. Each night I said what I was quite sure might be our last good-bye. I gathered up my heavy coat and scarf and hat and sought out a favorite LPN who was on duty and told her what I had done. Cissy is twenty years younger than I am but she was a mentor to my feelings through those last weeks. She gave me a warm embrace and assured me she would look in on my mother every few minutes and stay with her if she needed it.

"Do you want me to phone you if she is dying?" she asked. "Don't feel you have to say Yes; it is not an easy time often and it really sticks in your memories. You may want to remember her the way she lived." I thought for a moment and then I said, "Give me a call and I'll come."

That evening someone phoned and we talked for half an hour. As soon as we hung up, immediately the phone rang. "Your mother died a few minutes ago. It was very peaceful. Do you want to come over?"

"I'll be right there."

My mother's body was still warm as I kissed her. She looked as though she were simply asleep. She looked very peaceful—and while I was very choked with sadness, I was grateful that she, that we, had negotiated or navigated a way out of her Alzheimer's disease.

It is now seven or eight weeks later. Yesterday for the first time I was ready to sort through a lot of her papers. It was clear that as her capacity for making sense of her life diminished, my mother's solution was simple: she saved everything. From her journal that recorded receipt of her dividend checks, it was clear that her handwriting deteriorated quite suddenly in the winter and spring of her seventy-ninth year and by summer of that year the last entries were made.

There is much I regret about the disease and what a wasting it was of her in those years, but I am grateful too for the use we made of that time, salvaging so much even while we both were losing so much.

She died five years later. It seemed like an eternity, and I am sure it seemed even longer to her. But we had some of our most wonderful, most intimate times of being together and sharing in those last five years. There is much I regret about the disease and what a wasting it was of her in those years. But I am grateful too for the use we made of that time, salvaging so much even while we both were losing so much. Perhaps that is what all of life is, a salvaging even while we are losing. Alzheimer's disease just provides one context for doing that, and other people find other contexts. But finally it is all the same process, isn't it.

16.

Walking North

A Fascination with Maps

I remember being intrigued by maps when I was a boy. Treasure maps, topographical maps, military maps, maps of continents and maps of our town, they all fascinated me even though I wasn't lost and we had lived for almost all of my memory in our house. But maps located you, and whether big or small in scale a map represented your world, and by connecting the landmarks in sight with the cues printed on the map page, I had found a guide not only to the known worlds but to unknown ones.

A good riddle has to seem in some way
impossible, and yet you have to trust that
it is *not* impossible, and there is a good answer,
an adequate and satisfactory solution.

I also went through a riddle phase as a boy. I recall a map riddle that went like this: I walk twenty miles south, and then twenty miles east, and twenty miles north, and find that I have returned to the place I started out: where am I?

I don't recall whether I figured that out. Probably not. But I have always liked that riddle. Like all good riddles, it was so obvious once you cracked it, once you understood it. It was like the inner lights of the mind go on. I still remember the day as a boy when I realized that it was the daily newspaper which was "black and white and red all over." A good riddle has to have what I now call "cognitive dissonance" and yet be believable. It has to seem in some way impossible, and yet—this is what is required for believing a riddle has a good answer—you have to trust that it is *not* impossible and there is a good answer, an adequate and satisfactory solution.

For example, it is the notion of Earth having a North Pole which makes the Walking Riddle work. Only at the North Pole did all directions lead south, so that walking east when twenty miles south of the pole would be to walk the arc of a circle instead of walking the south side of a square of north, south, east and west. My young mind turned these things over and over. It was a fascination with the ways things were that did not wane until in adolescence I became aware of girls.

When Maps Begin to Fail Us

Now that I am in my late fifties I am still fascinated with my wife but I am taking on a renewed fascination with riddles. But the riddles are larger scale now and I find myself wondering if I can believe these riddles have good answers and "adequate" and "satisfactory" solutions.

Our family has come to the point in its generations that, like the complex arrangements of the gears in a grandfather's clock, it becomes clear that gear A is moved by Gear B, which in turn is on a spindle or axis with another gear—which, as it revolves, turns Gear C. Our children have graduated from college, starting out (as I recall our own starting out) on an adult life-trajectory of work and love and friction and relationships. *We* now are at the age I remember our parents being when we were married, now long ago. And of our own parents' generation, my mother was nearly the last.

With her Alzheimer's disease my mother seemed to keep on walking with us long after she was gone. Only the pulsing heart and warm hand lingered, reminding us of all the years this heart and this hand had been our companions, our help, sometimes our judge and jury and executioner, but always there for us in innumerable ways. For we were her children. Having her there was a part of what life is—or was. Everyone was someone's child even if we were grown, even if we were more or less estranged, even if we were a continent or more away. It went with the human map of the territory. It was a given, a fact of our existence.

In my forties and thirties I thought we all had our own life paths and each was different. Of course in many respects that is true. What I had not counted on was all these paths finally being drawn northward to the same omega point of death.

Life Paths That All Tend Northward

But now I realize we have all been slowly "walking north" together. No matter where we lived, someday a continent would no longer separate us. Yes, my mother, my father, my wife's parents who died before I was long in my wife's young life, all of them were walking a common path, a common direction, toward the north, toward our end point in this life.

I had known about the elderly that they sat wrapped in shawls and felt drafts and preferred to sit in high-backed armchairs with wings that protected them against winds and also could be snoozed in. But in my forties and thirties I thought we all had our own life paths and each was different. Of course in many respects that is true.

What I had not counted on was all these paths finally being drawn northward to the same omega point of death.

Yet just as metabolisms slow with age, and sleep seems to become somewhat more fitful, and people wake in the early-morning hours for trips to the bathroom they never knew they would need when they were younger, so there is a lot about the year after year life path which I had not thought about, in fact had not really needed to give much thought to.

But gradually "walking northward" came to summarize it all for me. We are walking, each of us, toward the North Pole. We are coming from every continent, every walk and station in life, and we all are doing it. The maps as drawn reflect that fact. We all know the North Pole as a symbol of dark and cold. It is only upon reflection, and perhaps some time with books or television or travel, that we come to realize the Arctic Circle (part way to the pole) is the map maker's convenience for noting that point beyond which in winter there is continuous darkness, a place where no sun shines. But this also notes the place where, in the brightness and warming of summer, the sun never sets and there is continual light. Take your pick: the map makers allow us to think in either way of what we are walking toward when we are walking northward. Are we going toward all-darkness or toward continual light?

Explorers All

My mother, my father, my mother-in-law and father-in-law, all who have gone before us, did just this—they preceded us. Before we were here, before we were born and arrived on this scene, it was their place. And by and large they leave it before we do. They are showing us the way—and that is the riddle.

If it really were simply a cartographer's trick, a map maker's conceit, the North Pole would matter less. But it is as though we all walked northward all our lives, perhaps veering east or west a bit, perhaps moving to Dallas or to San Diego or Minneapolis for a time, but always our lives tend northward. And at our end we all reach a point, as my boyhood riddle suggested, where if you can now only go northward, there is no more. And it ends. Your life ends. My father's life ends. My mother's life ends. My life ends.

When I contemplate the process by which our lives come to their completion and ending, I feel like I do when I hear accounts of the great explorers of the poles, Peary and Amundsen. It is an awesome accomplishment and it required so much help from so many. Yet it *has* been done. And it will now be done again. In fact each of us since birth has been set out upon this journey and exploration. We are explorers all. Some have greater vigor, some have the luck of greater resources or perhaps more congenial companions. But we all do it, and finally our trek "northward" becomes very personal and recognizably our own.

The riddle of our living and dying continues to grow in each of us.

As I say, I have always been fascinated with maps and riddles. As I have grown older the maps somehow have gotten less adequate and the riddles have become more all-encompassing. Perhaps that is what happens as you draw nearer to a complex end point or goal. It is as though life itself had a built-in magnetic deviation that shifts a bit each year until we learn to question our compasses even if we have not yet thrown them away. But whether we are ready or not, pages continue to be torn from the world's calendars, we each work our way further northward, and the riddle of our living and dying continues to grow in each of us.

Index

Quotations

Events, Names and Topics